ASSESSMENT AND INTERVENTION RESOURCE FOR HISPANIC CHILDREN

Clinical Competence Series

Series Editor
Robert T. Wertz, Ph.D.

ASSESSMENT AND INTERVENTION RESOURCE FOR HISPANIC CHILDREN

Hortencia Kayser, Ph.D.
New Mexico State University
Las Cruces

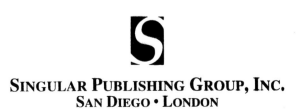

SINGULAR PUBLISHING GROUP, INC.
SAN DIEGO • LONDON

NOTICE TO THE READER

Publisher does not warrant or guarantee any of the products described herein or perform any independent analysis in connection with any of the product information contained herein. Publisher does not assume, and expressly disclaims, any obligation to obtain and include information other than that provided to it by the manufacturer.

The reader is expressly warned to consider and adopt all safety precautions that might be indicated by the activities herein and to avoid all potential hazards. By following the instructions contained herein, the reader willingly assumes all risks in connection with such instructions.

The Publisher makes no representation or warranties of any kind, including but not limited to, the warranties of fitness for particular purpose or merchantability, nor are any such representations implied with respect to the material set forth herein, and the publisher takes no responsibility with respect to such material. The publisher shall not be liable for any special, consequential, or exemplary damages resulting, in whole or part, from the readers' use of, or reliance upon, this material.

COPYRIGHT © 1998

Singular Publishing Group is a division of Thomson Learning. The Thomson Learning logo is a registered trademark used herein under license.

Printed in the United States of America
3 4 5 6 7 8 9 10 XXX 05 04

For more information, contact Singular Publishing Group, 401 West "A" Street, Suite 325 San Diego, CA 92101-7904; or find us on the World Wide Web at http://www.singpub.com

Library of Congress Cataloging-in-Publication Data:
ISBN: 1-5659-3750-3

CONTENTS

FOREWORD

com•pe•tence (kom'pə təns)   n.   The state or quality of being properly or well qualified; capable.

Clinicians crave competence. They pursue it through education and experience, through emulation and innovation. Some are more successful than others in attaining what they seek. This book, *Assessment and Intervention Resource for Bilingual Hispanic Children,* by Hortencia "Hart" G. Kayser opens the ever-increasing realm of Speech-Language Pathology in a bilingual setting. For many clinicians, this world is truly foreign. Dr. Kayser provides an introduction, orientation, and sensitivity that tells us where we are and what we need to do to provide essential services for bilingual Hispanic children. For the few clinicians who are experienced in bilingual Speech-Language Pathology, she extends their reach by providing specific methods for assessing, analyzing, and mending speech and language disorders in bilingual Hispanic children. Hart Kayser crosses borders and extends boundaries. Our attention to what she provides indicates our competence and our efforts to improve it, because competent clinicians seek competence as much for what it demands as for what it promises.

Robert T. Wertz, Ph.D.
Series Editor

PREFACE

When I was approached to organize this book as a resource manual for clinicians who work with bilingual populations, my first idea was to provide normative data for easy referencing. But as I spoke to clinicians, I found that what was also needed was a resource providing theoretical models. The quality of direct services to bilingual populations will be determined by the resources available to clinicians and agencies. The models that have been developed and proposed in this book will assist clinicians in their organization of services to children.

I have attempted to provide references that I have found useful and resources that may also provide additional information for serving children. The included examples and brief descriptions of assessment and intervention programs are not necessarily the only and best examples, but rather they are examples that can be improved upon depending on circumstances of the speech-language pathologist and the Hispanic population being served.

Much of the materials in the appendixes are used in our clinic at New Mexico State University, Las Cruces. As we continue to develop our services to Hispanic children and adults at NMSU, we will increase our efforts in helping speech-language pathologists with materials, handouts, and information.

ACKNOWLEDGMENTS

There are a number of people who have contributed time and effort in the production of this book. I would first like to thank a number of graduate students who spent long hours working on the manuscript tables, reviewing the literature in the library, and maneuvering through computer programs and websites. These students include Alisa Ball, Denise Bundy, Christine Hornak, Gloria Macias, Shelley Mondoux, Angelica Ortega, Roberta Player, Robert Quintana, Maria Trujillo, and Julie Webb. I am also grateful to all of the other bilingual graduate students with whom I have had the pleasure of learning from and working with through the years. I would also like to thank the Department of Special Education/Communication Disorders and the Office of the Vice President for Academic Affairs at New Mexico State University for supporting this project through graduate assistantships and work study student support.

CHAPTER

1

Hispanic Cultures

A Hispanic, as defined by the Census Bureau of the United States (Bureau of the Census, 1988), is an individual of Spanish background who may come from any race. To say that Hispanics have one culture would be an oversimplification of that definition, as Hispanics encompass a variety of cultures, just as they come from a variety of races. Hispanic, then, is a broad term used for convenience to identify individuals who come from a Spanish heritage and may or may not use Spanish as the language of the home.

This chapter reviews the literature of culture, demographics, family roles, and socialization. Perceptions of disabilities are also discussed.

I. THE HISPANIC POPULATION (Kayser, 1993; Langdon, 1992)

A. The United States has the fifth-largest Spanish-speaking population in the world, behind Mexico, Spain, Colombia, Argentina, and Peru.

B. Within the United States, the Hispanic population totaled 27 million in 1994, a 28% increase from the 1990 census.

   1. **It is projected that in the United States, Hispanics** will number 31 million by 2000 and 63 million by 2030.

   2. **Hispanic Groups:** Mexican Americans 58%; South and Central Americans 14%; Puerto Rican Americans 13%; Cuban Americans 6%.

   3. **The greatest proportion of Hispanics** are in California, Texas, New York, Florida, Illinois, Arizona, New Jersey, New Mexico, and Colorado.

      a. The 10 metropolitan areas with the greatest proportion of Hispanics are Laredo, TX; McAllen, TX; Brownsville, TX; El Paso, TX; Las Cruces, NM; Corpus Christi, TX, Santa Fe, NM; San Antonio, TX; Albuquerque, NM; and Pueblo, CO.

      b. The cities with the largest numbers are Los Angeles, New York, Miami, San Francisco, Chicago, Houston, San Antonio, El Paso, San Diego, and Dallas.

II. THE CONTEMPORARY HISPANIC

The U.S. Census (1996) confirms that there are differences in economic and educational attainment by the Hispanic population compared with the population as a whole. In general, Hispanics in the United States are likely to be less educated and to earn less income annually and are thus more likely to be below the poverty level than are non-Hispanics.

A. Fifty-three percent of Hispanics complete 4 years of high school with the rate among non-Hispanics 83%. The breakdown among Hispanics is:

   1. **Mexican Americans:** 45%

   2. **Puerto Rican Americans:** 51%

   3. **Cuban Americans:** 61%

   4. **Central and South Americans:** 64%

B. **Only 9% of Hispanics complete 4 or more years of college;** although among non-Hispanics, the rate is 23%. For Hispanics, the breakdown is:

   1. **Mexican Americans:** 7%

   2. **Puerto Rican Americans:** 10%

   3. **Cuban Americans:** 17%

   4. **Central and South Americans:** 17%

C. **The 1993 median income of Hispanic families** was $23,670, compared with $41,110 for non-Hispanic families.

   1. **Mexican Americans:** $19,970

   2. **Puerto Rican Americans:** $15,190

   3. **Cuban Americans:** $27,290

   4. **Central and South Americans:** $22,940

D. **About 27% of Hispanic families,** compared to 11% for non-Hispanic families, were living below the poverty level in 1996. The figures for individual populations are:

   1. **Mexican Americans:** 26%

   2. **Puerto Rican Americans:** 38%

   3. **Cuban Americans:** 14%

   4. **Central and South Americans:** 19%

E. **Hispanics have yet to experience the results of a truly equal society** that allows them to benefit from its educational and economic riches.

III. FAMILY AND SOCIALIZATION PRACTICES

Hispanic children are exposed to environments that are characterized by unique cultural beliefs and caregiving practices that are different from those of mainstream English-speaking populations (Garcia Coll, 1990). Primary among these practices is the Hispanic family's belief in the strength of the family.

A. Hispanic Cultural Tendencies

There are a number of cultural tendencies that have been reported in the literature concerning Hispanics. The following are descriptions that may not be universal to all Hispanics (N.B. Anderson & Battle, 1993; Kayser, 1993; Taylor, 1992).

1. **Members value nuclear and extended family.** The family is defined loosely with individuals able to become part of the family by being "compadrazimos" (a godparent).

2. **Members value family cohesion.** The family unity is paramount.

3. **There is respect for tradition** and traditional family and social roles.

4. **Members have a flexible sense of time.**

5. **There is close personal proximity during conversation.** Touching may be part of the interaction.

6. **Children and adults are not viewed as equal communication partners.** Children are expected to respect adult roles and not to consider themselves as equal to an adult.

7. **Children are encouraged to be independent learners.** Children are expected to observe and learn on their own.

8. **Children often participate in multiple-partner communication interactions.** Group interactions are encouraged as part of peer socialization.

B. Familism

Zayas and Palleja (1988) have employed this term for Puerto Rican home support for family integrity that gives shape and direction to the conduct of family members.

1. **Puerto Rican society** emphasizes the importance of the nuclear and extended family and cohesion among its members. Zayas and

Palleja (1988) state that the family governs the individual identities of its members and the collective identity of the family.

2. **The needs of the individual are considered secondary** to those of the family.

3. **The family reputation is a central consideration** in an individual's action.

4. ***Respeto y Obediencia*** (respect and obedience) are stressed, with the greatest respect for grandparents.

5. **Members learn to accept** these responsibilities to preserve family integrity, tradition, and social and emotional equilibrium.

6. **There are specific qualities** that Hispanics may observe in their relationships. These include *respeto* (respect), *dignidad* (dignity), *personalismo* (personalism), *honor* (honor), and *confianza* (trust) (Harry, 1992).

   a. These qualities transcend social class.

   b. The focus is on the inner importance of a person, uniqueness of a person—the person's goodness, or worth.

7. **Relationships are important:** Networking among community members and extended families make up a community as a system of trustworthy individuals.

C. **Heath (1986) describes Mexican-American** families as either open or closed to the mainstream culture.

   1. **Closed:** the children within the family are protected and, to some extent, isolated from the mainstream. The children do not have the opportunity to learn about mainstream values and communication functions.

   2. **Open:** the children participate in the community through secondary institutions, such as public libraries and the Boy Scouts.

   3. **The mother's level of formal education** was a factor in the type of teaching strategies she used with her children according to Laosa (1978).

a. The higher the mother's level of formal education, the more she used inquiry and praise as teaching strategies.

b. The lower the mother's level of formal education, the more she used modeling as a teaching strategy and for boys, in particular, the more the mother appeared to control and punish physically.

4. **Parental emphasis on observation and independence in learning** was discovered by Valdes (1986).

a. It is assumed that children are able to judge when they are ready to undertake a task and their performance is the best that they are able to do at the chosen time.

b. Adults provide guidance if it is needed or requested, but the parent rarely offers much in the way of unsolicited verbal instructions.

IV. PERCEPTIONS OF DISABILITIES

The common basis for the belief system of many is Catholic theological ideology. Mexican Catholic ideology includes Indian practices, but Cuban and Puerto Rican Catholicism may include African religious beliefs, for example, Yoruba, which is sometimes called *santerismo* or *espiritismo* (Harry, 1992). The following are commonly reported beliefs about disabilities (P. P. Anderson & Fenichel, 1989; Hanline & Daley, 1992; Langdon, 1992; Maestas & Erickson, 1992; Meyerson, 1983; Roseberry-McKibbin, 1995).

A. **"Evil eye" or "mal ojo"** is obtained by admiring an individual or envying the person giving that person illness. *Curanderos,* medicine women, are called to perform rituals, give prayers, and provide herbal medicinal teas to counteract the evil that affected the afflicted individual.

B. **Susto** is a severe scare to a child that might cause the child to begin stuttering.

C. **A full moon or an eclipse** will cause a cleft palate in an unborn child, if the mother views this without the typical remedy of a safety pin under her clothes to protect the child.

D. *Curanderismo,* folk medicine using herbs, prayers, and rituals to heal all illnesses, may be practiced.

E. Institutionalization may be resisted by the family. Families will take care of their own children and elderly and may not use public facilities to care for their ill family members.

F. Parents may believe that they are being punished for wrongdoing. A past sin may be blamed for a child having a disability.

G. Catholic parents may accept disabilities stoically. Parents may believe that God has given the family a cross to bear, and they accept the difficulties that confront the family.

H. Some families may hide a disabled child, if the family takes pride in their health and vitality.

I. Children with disabilities may be indulged by family and friends. Family members may not have the typical role expectations for a child with disability and thus allow him or her to have more freedom and less structure than a typical child.

J. Children with disabilities may not be expected to participate in treatment and their own care. An explanation may be that since the child is a gift from God, the child should not be changed from what God has ordained.

K. Invisible disabling conditions may not be accepted. In Mexico, learning disability is not an accepted concept. Teacher failure and, more commonly, student laziness are used as explanations for the children who do not succeed in academics.

L. Some families may use spiritualists to seek healing and dispel evil spirits.

V. CONCLUSION

The Hispanic population in the United States is a heterogeneous group composed of many different cultures and races. The Spanish language is the one commonality for these groups, but the language will vary according to respective dialects. The backgrounds, experiences, political views, education, and beliefs about the mainstream culture are just a few of the many variables that will affect the interactions between this population and the professions of speech-language pathology and audiology. Being aware of these differences is just the beginning of developing sensitive service provision. Understanding and knowledge about these groups are required for appropriate assessment and treatment of communication impairments.

CHAPTER

2

Bilingual Education

Bilingual education for students from culturally and linguistically diverse groups has been a controversial and political topic. The issues that surround the language of instruction and bilingual education have been discussed in terms of legal, political, social, economic, and cultural ramifications for three decades. This type of education allows a student to use his or her home language as part of the educational process. It has been documented as effective for students whose home language is not English (Hakuta, 1986). This chapter discusses the myths of bilingual education, defines bilingual education as it has evolved through the decades, lists variables in effective bilingual education programs, and discusses issues that must be part of the evaluation for effectiveness. Also included in this chapter is a summary of research on bilingual education and an explanation of English as a second language (ESL) programs.

I. BILINGUAL EDUCATION: CHARGES AND REBUTTALS

There have been a number of myths concerning bilingual education that have continued to be repeated among teachers, parents, and public policy makers.

These myths have affected the general public's understanding of the effectiveness of bilingual education. Following are the more common myths. Hakuta (1986) calls these "charges" and he provides rebuttals.

A. There Is No Historical Basis for Bilingual Education.

There has been bilingual education in the United States since the country was founded.

B. Bilingual Education Lacks Popular Support

Canvassing of bilingual communities indicates that bilingual education is supported for assistance provided to children in learning English and other academic subjects.

C. Most Bilingual Programs Are Maintenance Not Transitional Models

Bilingual education is mandated as transitional in programming. Maintenance programs are expensive and are not supported by local school districts.

D. Young Children Learn a Second Language Quickly, Anyway

Children do learn a second language quickly, but lose their ability to speak the native language more rapidly than older children. Thus, there are cognitive detrimental effects when children lose their ability to function in the home language while learning the second language.

E. Valuable Time for Learning in English Is Wasted

Children who are provided academic instruction in the native language while learning English do as well on English language tests as children who are taught only in English.

F. Bilingual Education Is Not Effective

Bilingual education programs across the country have been found to be effective in educating children and maintaining these children's progress through graduation.

G. There Are not as Many Children Who Are LEPs (Limited English Proficient) as Expected

Each school district defines which children are LEP. Some school systems do not offer services to children who need services, because of a strict definition of limited English proficient.

II. LANGUAGE OF INSTRUCTION WITH BILINGUAL CHILDREN

There has been considerable debate concerning the language of instruction for minority language children in the United States. Currently, the debate is focused on children with speech and language impairments from a non-English-speaking background. This debate has caused some confusion by the general public about the relative effectiveness of English-only instruction versus native-language instruction. This confusion may stem from the different bilingual education systems that are found in the United States and Canada. Therefore, a description of the two systems is warranted.

A. Immersion Bilingual Education

Many Canadian programs are "additive" immersion bilingual education programs. Majority language children who speak English enter kindergarten classrooms that are taught in French, the minority language (Fradd & Tikunoff, 1987; Hakuta, 1986). As the children progress through the grade levels, they are increasingly exposed to English, the home language, until they are receiving half of their education in English and half in French.

1. The goal of these programs is to maintain the home language, while helping children to acquire a valued second language. There are four important sociocultural features of such additive immersion programs:

    a. They are intended for children from the majority group language (i.e., English);

    b. Teachers and administrators value and support the children's home language and culture;

    c. The child and parents value their home language and culture; and

d. Acquisition of the second language is regarded as a positive skill by the participants and parents (McLaughlin, 1985).

2. The success of additive immersion bilingual education programs is believed to be due in large part to the four sociocultural features. Programs that share such features are found in target schools in major cities in the United States and throughout Canada and are considered to be enrichment programs for majority language children (Hakuta, 1986).

3. Research supports the effectiveness of additive immersion (Lambert & Tucker, 1972; Swain & Barik, 1978).

B. The United States Has Varied Curriculum Designs

These include (Fradd & Tikunoff, 1987):

1. **The maintenance model** designed to develop bilingualism and biliteracy;

2. **The transitional model** designed to use the non-English language to facilitate the learning of English through curriculum content;

3. **The English as a second language** (ESL) model, which is usually a component of the first two models; and

4. **The high-intensity model** found in middle and high schools, where students are expected to learn English rapidly.

C. The effectiveness of transitional bilingual education in the United States has not been documented adequately (Hakuta, 1986; McLaughlin, 1985) as contrasted to Canada.

1. Thus, there is the opinion that immersion should be used at least partially with minority language children in the U.S., because it has been documented to be effective in Canada.

2. Neither transitional bilingual education nor immersion will be effective with minority language children in the United States states Hakuta (1986). As long as education is a subtractive rather than an additive experience—one of assimilation at all cost—and without respect for a child's home language and culture, minority language children will not succeed in either model. This makes common

sense especially for children who are having difficulty acquiring their first language.

III. U.S. LEGISLATION

A. Transitional Bilingual Education Is the Model Mandated by the Elementary and Secondary Education Act

This act is also known as the Bilingual Education Act (BEA) (1968). In addition, transitional bilingual education is supported by the *Lau v. Nichols* (1974) U.S. Supreme Court decision. Minority language students are to be instructed in their home language until they are able to receive exclusive instruction in English (Hakuta, 1986). These children receive instruction in the home language beginning in kindergarten, and as they progress through the grades, they are increasingly exposed to the majority language (English). Once these children are determined to have adequate proficiency in English, they are transferred to English-only instruction. The home language is not maintained.

B. Education Amendments of 1974

Reauthorized and revised Bilingual Education Act (BEA) (Chamot, 1988; Cummins, 1995; Skutnabb-Kangas, 1995).

1. Authorization of new grants for state education agencies; technical assistance; training programs separate from instructional programs; and a national clearing house to collect, analyze, and disseminate information on bilingual education programs.

2. Bilingual education programs **defined** as instruction given in, with study of, English necessary for a child to progress effectively through the educational system. The native language was to be used only to allow the children to progress in academic subjects while acquiring English.

3. Voluntary enrollment, to a limited degree, authorized for English-speaking children in bilingual education programs.

4. Teaching a foreign language to English-speaking children discouraged. (This reinforced a focus on English language development and fostered neglect of native language development.)

5. Funding banned for two-way bilingual education programs (minority children learning English as a second language and majority children learning minority language as a second language).

C. Education Amendments 1978

Reauthorized and revised the Bilingual Education Act, and expanded the scope and size of the program.

1. Funding increased, with annual increases;

2. New grant programs authorized;

3. A commission of education formed to collect and publish information on a wide range of issues relating to language minority students, as well as providing a definition of bilingual education;

4. Eligibility was clarified. Limited English proficient (LEP) supplanted limited English speaking to recognize the importance of reading and writing, understanding, and cognitive skills, in addition to speaking (which reinforced the deficit approach to education);

5. Voluntary enrollment was clarified, with specification that up to 40% of the students can be non-English speakers to prevent the segregation of children on the basis of national origin; and

6. The ban on programs designed to teach foreign languages was eliminated.

D. Title VI of Civil Rights Act of 1964

1. Prohibited discrimination on basis of race, color, or national origin in federally assisted programs and activities and imposed grant-making agencies with the responsibility for ensuring compliance;

2. Office of Civil Rights (OCR) was established in Department of Health, Education, and Welfare (DHEW)

E. DHEW General Guidelines, 1968

In 1968, DHEW issued general guidelines which held schools responsible for assuring that students of a particular race, color, or national origin are not denied opportunity to education generally available to other students in the system.

F. Memorandum, 1970

In 1970, a memorandum was issued from OCR that gave specific information on responsibilities of school districts whose national origin minority enrollments exceeded 5%.

1. Prohibited the assignment of minority students to classes for the mentally retarded on the basis of criteria that essentially measure or evaluate English language skills and stopped denial of access to college preparation courses on a basis directly related to the failure of the school system to teach English language skills.

2. Specified that ability grouping and any tracking system must meet language skills needs as early as possible and must not operate as an educational dead-end or permanent track.

3. Required that schools must adequately notify minority group parents of school activities therefore, the notice should be provided in a language other than English.

G. Unenacted 1982 Bilingual Education Act (BEA) Amendments

1. Elimination of the requirement that BEA-funded programs make some instructional use of a LEP student's native language was a primary change sought.

2. No action was taken on the legislation in the 97th Congress, despite public testimony and expert evidence that contradicted the administrative position on English-only instruction.

H. 1984 Bilingual Education Act Amendments

1. Education and language-minority groups provided help in developing the legislation to reauthorize and revise the act which led to strengthened and expanded BEA legislation.

2. Had primary goal extended to all BEA programs to enable LEP children to achieve competence in English and to meet grade promotion and graduation standards.

3. Required all BEA programs to provide LEP students with intensive structured English language instruction.

4. Replaced the single, basic BEA grant for programs with several programs. For example, family English literacy programs for adults and out-of-school youth were enabled, plus special preschool, special education and gifted and talented programs for LEP students. Bilingual programs of demonstrated academic excellence were identified.

5. Two general purpose instructional programs were authorized: Transition bilingual education received 75% of the funding and dual bilingual education (DBE) was also set up.

6. Legislation specified that DBE must enable LEP students not only to become proficient in English and to meet grade promotion and graduation requirements, but also to become proficient in the native language.

7. Where possible, DBE programs were to enroll near equal numbers of native English-speaking children and children whose native language is the second language of instruction and study.

8. A compromise that authorized a third category of general instruction grants—special alternative instructional programs (SAIP), or monolingual English programs. There was no instruction for the students in their native language.

   a. For some school districts, establishing DBE was administratively impractical because there were too few students with a particular home language

   b. Qualified personnel shortages hampered implementation in some cases.

I. Education Amendments of 1988

1. Removed restrictions on the amount of BEA funds that could be devoted to English-only SAIP programs.

2. Programs supported by Title VII, 1988.

   a. **Basic bilingual programs.** Financial assistance provided to local school systems to implement educational program designed to assist LEP children to improve their English language skills; provided for supplementary activities for parents and teachers of children in programs.

b. **Demonstration projects.** Sought to demonstrate outstanding programs of bilingual education. Priorities for funding were allocated to projects serving activities and projects with outstanding approaches for developing participation of English-speaking children.

c. **Bilingual vocational instructor training program.** Bilingual vocational training provided to persons whose dominant language was not English and who were either unemployed or underemployed because of their limited English-speaking ability.

d. **Bilingual vocational instructor training program.** Provides training to persons to improve their skills and qualifications as vocational education instructors to LEP persons.

e. **State educational agency projects for coordinating technical assistance.** Assists bilingual education programs within a state by disseminating information, facilitating information exchanges among programs and aiding program planning in general.

f. **Bilingual education service centers.** Provides training in bilingual education to persons working in a bilingual education program and to parents of children in a bilingual program.

g. **Evaluation, dissemination, and assessment centers.** Assesses, evaluates, and disseminates bilingual education materials for use in bilingual education programs.

h. **Materials development centers.** Develop instructional and testing materials for use in bilingual education programs.

i. **Training projects.** Train existing or future bilingual teachers, parents, and others in bilingual education.

j. **School of Education projects (Dean's grants).** Provides programs at accredited universities or colleges that lead to degrees in bilingual-bicultural education.

k. **Fellowship programs.** Provides financial assistance to full-time graduate students who are preparing to become bilingual teacher trainers.

l. **Refugee Education Assistance Act of 1980.** Supports awards for financial assistance to state educational agencies for distribution among local schools providing supplementary education services to refugee children enrolled in public and private schools.

m. **Bilingual desegregation support programs.** Provide financial assistance to local school systems to help meet the educational needs of children from non-English-speaking homes and who lack equal educational opportunity because of language and culture.

n. **Research agenda.** Provides funds for research in bilingual education.

IV. LAU v. NICHOLS (FULL SIGNIFICANCE OF OFFICE OF CIVIL RIGHTS, 1970 TITLE VI)

A. The Case

1. The OCR memorandum (See item F.) was not realized until 1974, when the U.S. Supreme Court handed down its first and only substantive decision about the legal responsibilities of schools serving LEP students, *Lau v. Nichols.*

2. *Lau v. Nichols* was a class action suit by parents of nearly 3,000 Chinese pupils among 16,500 students in San Francisco public school system; two thirds of the Chinese pupils had received no English assistance.

3. The San Francisco Board of Education was directed to rectify the problems of Chinese students.

4. The Supreme Court found the school district in violation of Title VI, but declined to rule on constitutional claims by the plaintiffs.

B. Lau Remedies of 1975

1. DHEW began to develop remedial rather than compliance guidelines for districts not in compliance with Title VI under Lau.

2. Lau remedies specified proper approaches, methods, and procedures for:

   a. Identifying and evaluating minority students' English language skills;

   b. Determining appropriate instructional treatments;

   c. Deciding when LEP students were ready for mainstream classes; and

   d. Determining the proficiency standards to be met by teachers of language minority children.

3. Elementary schools were generally required to provide LEP students with English as a second language instruction as well as academic subject matter instruction in a student's strongest language until the student achieved enough proficiency in English to effectively learn in a monolingual English classroom.

4. Three instructional models were specified for schools. All required the use of a student's native language and cultural factors in instruction.

   a. **Transitional model:** Native language instruction was provided only until students became fully functional in English.

   b. **Bicultural-bilingual model:** ongoing instruction and development of both English and native language resulting in students being capable of functioning in both languages and cultures.

   c. **Multilingual-multicultural model:** providing instruction and development of English and, at best, two other languages.

   d. Table 2–1 provides a description of bilingual programs for Canada and the United States (S. H. Fradd & Tikunoff, 1987).

V. EDUCATIONAL RESEARCH

Recent research findings from many parts of the world show clearly that maintaining and developing the native language (L1) by using it as a medium of instruction for a major part of the school day has no negative effects on the development of the second language (L2) and, in many cases, has very

Table 2–1. Description of Bilingual Programs

Program	Government Policy	Parents' Status and Views
Immersion in Canada	Enhancement of bilingualism and multiculturalism. Promotion of international economic advantage.	Additive-middle class. Parents initiate and support the program. Students' skills in both languages are valued.
Transitional Programs in the United States	No clear policy for bilingualism. Bilingualism is not viewed as an advantage but is difficult to maintain.	Programs are viewed as remedial. Generally, bilingualism may be considered as an advantage, but is difficult to maintain.
Other models in the United States	Flexibility at the local level; bilingualism is viewed as an advantage.	Socioeconomic status is generally low. Parent participation is generally promoted, but in actuality parents have little to say. There may be exceptions, however.

Note: L1, first language; L2, second language; CALP, cognitive academic language proficiency; BICS, basic interpersonal communication skills

Source: From *Bilingual Education and Bilingual Special Education: A Guide for Administrators* (p. 36), by S. H. Fradd and W. J. Tikunoff, 1987, Austin, TX: PRO-ED. Copyright 1987 by PRO-ED. Adapted with permission.

positive effects, both on the development of L2 and other academic skills (Cummins, 1979, 1980). Bilingual children often do poorly at school and many experience emotional conflicts. Some researchers and administrators have seized on the obvious scapegoat and blamed children's failure on their bilingualism. Children may be made to feel that it is necessary to reject the home culture and frequently may be unable to identify fully with either cultural group. But, many research studies suggest that bilingual children who develop their proficiency in both languages have intellectual and academic

Teachers	Curriculum
All teachers are bilingual. Has the support from the community and administrators. Are offered a uniform preparation.	Students are expected to use both languages. All students begin at the same level of L2. Literacy in both languages is emphasized. Both languages have the same value. No real transition in programs.
Only some teachers are bilingual. May have community and administrator support. Training institutions offer great variation in preparation. Requires large numbers of bilingual teachers. Many rely on teacher aides.	Use of L1 until L2 is mastered. Students need to catch up to function in an all-English curriculum. Transition to English is often made. When surface language skills (BICS) are judged adequate. Some other programs may transition students when sufficient (CALP) skills are acquired.
Only some teachers are bilingual. May have community and administrator support. Training institutions offer great variation in preparation. Requires fewer bilingual teachers. Use of language grouping. More emphasis on teacher cooperation.	Use of L1 and L2 is acquired. L1 is valued. Provision is made for uniformity in language instruction. Transition to English is done only when student has higher language skills in L1 (CALP).

advantages over monolingual children (Hakuta, 1986). It just makes sense that a high level of proficiency in two languages is likely to be an intellectual advantage for children in all subjects across the curriculum, when compared with monolingual classmates. In social situations where there is likely to be serious erosion of the first (minority) language, there is a need for the development and maintenance of that language to prevent intellectual performance from suffering. Different forms of educational programs should be available to meet the needs of students from varying linguistic backgrounds.

A. Classroom Organization and Development of Bilingualism (Wong-Fillmore, 1989)

1. Open classroom structure (i.e., children are allowed to work at various study centers at their own pace) works only if there are enough native speakers of the target language to provide necessary, sustained interactions with L2 learners.

2. Classrooms with large numbers of L2 learners require more teacher-centered structuring (i.e., teacher is controlling the language and learning input) to ensure adequate input.

3. Conditions for additive process in bilingualism is building L2 on an L1 foundation. Conditions for the process are:

    a. The family language is valued and both languages are used for a variety of purposes.

    b. Bilingualism is promoted at home and school and is socially advantageous.

    c. Learners have well-developed L1 before L2 learning begins.

    d. Learners have opportunity to develop literacy in L1 and L2.

    e. Learning takes place where there are many opportunities to interact with L2 speakers.

    f. L2 speakers are willing to help L1 speakers.

    g. L1 speakers receive appropriate instructional and corrective support for English use.

4. Subtractive bilingualism has L2 replacing L1. Conditions for the process are:

    a. There is great pressure to learn English.

    b. Family language does not function in the social world.

    c. The younger the child, the greater the loss of L1 when exposed to L2.

>   **d.** Language learning takes place in settings where learners greatly outnumber speakers of English.
>
>   **e.** English-speaking role models are inexperienced in English.
>
>   **f.** Learners of English do not get adequate instruction in English or feedback.

5. Criteria for bicultural equilibrium (Baetens-Beardsmore, 1986):

>   **a.** Positive parental attitudes towards bilingualism.
>
>   **b.** Bilingual-bicultural education.
>
>   **c.** Monolingual and cultural references are evaluated so as not to bias one culture.
>
>   **d.** Teachers should be native speakers of respective languages with positive attitudes towards both languages.

B. Variables Leading to Effective Bilingual Education (Cummins, 1995)

1. Bilingual and bilingual-trained teachers.

2. Bilingual materials.

3. Appropriate pupil material content.

4. Low student anxiety level (supportive, nonauthoritarian environments).

5. High student internal motivation that is not focused on the use of L2.

6. High self-confidence (fair chance to succeed, high teacher expectations).

7. Adequate linguistic development in L1 (L1 taught well).

8. Sufficiently relevant, cognitively demanding subject matter provided.

9. Opportunity to develop L1 outside school in linguistically demanding formal contexts.

10. L2 teaching supports and does not harm L1 development.

11. Adequate linguistic development in L2 (taught well).

12. L2 input adapted to pupils' L2 level.

13. Opportunity to practice L2 in peer group contexts.

14. Exposure to native speaker L2 use in linguistically demanding formal contexts.

VI. A QUESTIONNAIRE FOR TEACHER AND PROGRAM EFFECTIVENESS

Teacher expectations of children's potential for academic success and children's true potential can be overlooked, but low expectations can be damaging. This can be reduced through staff development with open discussions and questionnaires (Maybin, 1985). Crucial questions are:

A. Are all staff aware of the language and dialect repertoires of the pupils in the school?

B. Do staff members recognize that pupils' abilities to use language effectively have an important impact on their view of themselves and, therefore, on their confidence as learners?

C. Do staff accept the validity of all pupils' spoken abilities and use of these as a basis for developing their skills in reading and writing?

D. Are staff knowledgeable about what is meant by dialect, and do they have a positive approach to dialects different from the standard? How is this reflected in the way they assess pupils' written work?

E. Are staff knowledgeable about the native tongues that their pupils speak and do they see these as having a potential for good or a real strength in the school?

F. What different cultures are represented within your school?

G. How is this diversity reflected in the character of the school?

H. How does the school give value to the special experiences that culturally different children can offer?

I. How do children and staff learn about important cultural practices of the cultures represented in the school?

J. What are the different perceptions of the educational and social norms in the cultures represented in your school?

K. How does your school presently respond to overt racist behavior among staff and children (name calling, denigratory comments about other cultures, physical assaults, stereotyping, deliberate mispronunciation of names, etc.)?

L. Does the school acknowledge and support pupils' bilingualism and promote an interest in their language among all pupils?

M. Is there a satisfactory system within the school for identifying pupils who need help with English as their second language, for providing this help, and for monitoring progress?

N. Are the teaching resources for English as a second language sufficient to meet the needs of the pupils in the school, and are they organized so that pupils have access to them in a range of subject matter?

O. Do teachers make positive attempts to bring out the experience of pupils who as yet are not entirely confident in expressing themselves in English?

P. Has progress been made in responding to the issue of language diversity through the language policy and practice of the whole school?

Q. How is the use of community languages promoted in your school?

R. What provisions are made for the formal learning of community languages?

S. If there are formal language classes, how are they organized?

T. How does your school support community efforts for native language maintenance?

VII. CONCERNS FOR PARENTS

Bilingualism in the home, whether the language of the home is the same or different from the language of the school, matters very little in comparison to the quality of the interaction children experience with adults (Corson, 1990).

A. The success of many groups of children under home-school language switch conditions (e.g., French immersion) shows that concepts developed in L1 in the home can readily be transferred to L2 in school.

B. If minority parents attempt to use L2 in the home, the quality of interaction between parents and children will often suffer.

C. Parents not proficient in L2 are likely to expose their children to an inadequate L2 model and to spend less time interacting with them.

D. Teachers should encourage parents to promote the development of L1 through such activities as telling or reading stories to their children and generally spending time with them.

VIII. SECOND LANGUAGE TEACHING

There are a number of approaches or methods to the teaching of English as a second language (ESL). Children are taught English within the primary classroom or may be pulled out of the classroom for varied times to teach them English. Usually, ESL does not include academic instruction and is not considered part of bilingual education. The following are brief explanations of different approaches (Larsen-Freeman, 1986). See Figure 2–1 for a form for use to document a student's language dominance and proficiency.

Name: _____ Grade: _____ Age: _____

School: _____ Teacher: _____ Room: _____

Length of Residency in the U.S.: _____ Country of Origin: _____

Program Placement: Ed. _____ Bil. Ed. _____ ESL _____ Migrant Ed. _____ Other _____

If appropriate, percentage of English instruction _____ Native language instruction _____ ESL _____

Grades in bil. ed. program (circle those that apply: Preschool K 1 2 3 4 5 6 7 8 9 10 11 12

Grades in ESL program (circle those that apply): Preschool K 1 2 3 4 5 6 7 8 9 10 11 12

A. Language Use

    1. Home Language Survey: Date _____

        1. _____ First language learned by student

        2. _____ Language most frequently used by student at home

        3. _____ Language most frequently used by parents with student

        4. _____ Language most frequently used by adults with each other at home

        5. _____ Language most frequently used by student with siblings

    Based on the above, indicate primary home language:

    English _____   Other language _____   Both _____

    2. Observation of relative language usage (to be completed by a bilingual observer):

    Observer(s) _____ Date(s) of Observation _____

Check (✓) the language(s) the student uses with monolingual and bilingual individuals in each of the following contexts. If the student's language is characterized by code switching, place a "C" beside the check (✓).

Contexts	Only English *M	B	Mostly English M	B	Equal Use M	B	Mostly Other M	B	Only Other M	B
1. Informal with peers (playground, cafeteria, bus, etc.)										
2. Informal with adults (hallways, play areas, cafeteria, off-campus)										
3. Formal with peers (classroom, lab, library, etc.)										
4. Formal with adults (classroom, lab, library, etc.)										
Number of checks in each column (✓)										
Number of checks involving code switching (✓ C)										

*M = With monolingual speakers   B = With bilingual individuals

Based on the above, the most frequent used language is:

English _____ Other language _____ Both _____

Comments: _____

Figure 2–1. Profile of language dominance and proficiency

A. Grammar-Translation Method

This approach teaches language through literacy. The students read passages and answer questions about the readings. Other activities include memorizing grammar rules and memorizing native language equivalents of the target language vocabulary.

B. Direct Method

This process has students perceive meaning directly through use of the target language. Pantomime and visual aids are used to exemplify key concepts. Students speak the language and communicate in real-life situations. Grammar is learned inductively.

C. Audio-lingual Method

In this method, the learner repeats patterns until she or he is able to produce them spontaneously. Once patterns are learned, the speaker can substitute words to make new sentences. The teacher directs and controls students' learning.

D. The Silent Way

This approach focuses on students' development of their own inner criteria for correctness. Reading, writing, speaking, and listening are all used for learning. Teachers remain silent to help the student develop self-reliance and initiative. The students do most of the talking and interacting as the teacher arranges the situations for language learning.

E. Sugestopedia

The learning environment is relaxed and subdued, with low lighting and soft music in the background. Students imagine being a person within the culture. Dialogs are presented and students relax and listen to these with appropriate background music.

F. Community Language Learning

Teachers recognize that learning can be threatening and thus understand and accept students' fears. Teachers help students feel secure and overcome these fears. The students choose what they want to learn to say in the target language.

G. Total Physical Response Method

There is a primary emphasis placed on listening comprehension. Students demonstrate comprehension by acting out commands issued by the teacher. Activities are designed to be fun and to allow students to assume active learning roles. Activities include games and skits.

H. The Communicative Approach

This approach stresses the need to teach communicative competence as opposed to linguistic competence. Functions are emphasized over forms. Students work with materials in small groups on communicative activities and practice in negotiating meaning.

IX. CONCLUSION

Bilingual education is an immediate need for children who are learning English as a second language. Bilingual education is effective when educators are knowledgeable about the philosophy and pedagogy for helping minority language children develop cognitively and linguistically. Speech-language pathologists and audiologists need to be aware of the contributions of this form of education and its importance to Hispanic children in the United States. All children who enter our schools have the right to receive an education. The focus should not be on teaching English, but rather on educating young minds in the language(s) that will foster academic growth and development.

CHAPTER

3

Bilingualism

Haugen (1953) provided two premises that continue to ring true among minority language speakers in the United States: (a) necessity is the mother of bilingualism and (b) the only common thing about bilinguals is that they are not monolingual. This chapter provides definitions of bilingualism, variables that affect the bilingualism of an individual, universals among bilingual speakers, and a summary of the research on second language acquisition.

I. BILINGUALISM DEFINED

Baetens-Beardsmore (1986) has stated that definitions of bilingualism have continued to be offered without a feeling of some progress in this area. The term bilingualism has different meanings for different individuals. It has been defined with varying degrees of strictness, depending on how proficient or competent a speaker must be to be considered bilingual. It becomes imperative to define "bilingual" every time the term is used.

A. Bloomfield (1935) defines bilingual as an individual who has native-like control of two languages and exhibits no loss of the native language.

B. Thiery (1976) describes *ambilingual ability* as characteristic of only the true bilingual. Ambilingualism is rare.

C. MacNamara's (1967) definition states that a bilingual individual possesses at least one of the language skills in the two languages to a minimal degree (listening, speaking, reading, or writing).

D. Skutnabb-Kangas (1995) states "A speaker is bilingual who is able to function in two (or more) languages either in monolingual or bilingual communities in accordance with the sociocultural demands made on an individual's communicative and cognitive competence by these communities and by the individual herself or himself, at the same level as native speakers and who is able positively to identify with both (or all) language groups (and cultures) as parts of them (p. 46)."

E. Hundreds of Other Definitions

Definitions can be organized by:

1. **Origin.** A speaker is bilingual who:

   a. Has learned two languages in the family from native speakers from birth.

   b. Has used two languages in parallel as a means of communication from birth.

2. **Competence.** A speaker is bilingual who:

   a. Has mastery of two languages.

   b. Has native-like control of two languages.

   c. Has equal mastery of two languages.

   d. Can produce complete, meaningful utterances in two or more languages.

   e. Has at least some knowledge and control of structure of two or more languages.

   f. Has come into contact with another language.

3. **Function.** A speaker is bilingual who uses (or can use) two languages (in most situations in accordance with self-wishes and the demands of the community).

4. **Identification.** A speaker is bilingual who:

   a. Internally self-identifies as bilingual with two languages and/or two cultures (or parts of them).

   b. Externally identified by others as bilingual as a native speaker of two languages.

II. A TYPOLOGY

Baetens-Beardsmore (1986) summarized a typology of bilingualism that helps assist professionals who must classify or describe how an individual acquired a second language. Each of these typologies describes the bilingual individual in broad terms, but they do not address proficiency levels for each of the languages. He describes eight types of bilinguals.

A. Ambilingual

One who has language abilities like the monolingual in each language. This person has form, content, and use abilities that are equal to those of monolinguals who are the same age and intelligence level. This person does not make "mistakes" in either language, and no one would be able to detect that this individual spoke a second language. This level of proficiency is rare.

B. Equilingual

Person with balanced proficiency in the two languages, but the linguistic skills are not like monolinguals in either language. If the equilingual speaks language A or B, the monolingual speakers of that language would recognize that the individual is a speaker of another language. This is the most common type of bilingual.

C. Semilingual

Individual who has retarded development in both languages. Baetens-Beardsmore (1986) suggests that this term has outlived its usefulness in the research literature, because there has not been any empirical investigation to support this type of bilingualism.

D. Incipient

One who is beginning to make sense of the second language, either receptively or expressively. An individual usually becomes a receptive incipient bilingual and then an expressive incipient bilingual.

E. Passive, or Receptive

Person with comprehension of a second language.

F. Active, or Expressive

Individual has active use of both languages.

G. Academic

One has learned the second language through classroom instruction, such as in high school or college courses.

H. Natural

Person has learned the second language through circumstances, such as one language is spoken at home and the second in school. The majority of Hispanic children learn the second language because of circumstances, for example, elementary classrooms.

III. SOCIETAL FACTORS AFFECTING BILINGUALISM

The community may have many societal factors that are relevant to the individual's bilingualism. These societal factors will determine whether the community will be *stable* in the use of the two languages over several generations or *transitional*, meaning that the community will consist of monolingual English speakers within two generations (Sanchez, 1983). These societal factors include whether the minority language population is:

A. Immigrant-based or Indigenous

B. Of Recent Origin or Long-standing

C. Greater in number in relation to the majority language speakers

D. Evenly distributed within the community

E. Urban or Rural

F. Near or far from the native tongue country

G. Frequently visiting the native tongue country (Baetens-Beardsmore, 1986; N. Miller, 1984).

IV. UNIVERSALS

A. Transitional Versus Stable Bilingualism

Individuals can be in transition from monolingualism in Spanish to monolingualism in English. The stable bilingual speaker is one who maintains both languages. The following is an explanation of the continuum.

   1. AA is a monolingual speaker of Spanish

   2. Ab is a speaker of Spanish who understands English.

   3. AB is an active speaker of English and Spanish.

   4. Ba is a speaker of English who understands Spanish.

   5. A is a monolingual speaker of English.

   6. Continuum: A—Ab—AB—Ba—B.

   7. An individual may move through this continuum in one generation or maintain the active use of both languages for life.

B. Transference (Interference)

Transference is the observable element of marked bilingual speech. Originally, interference meant the use of formal elements of one code within the context of another, that is, phonological, morphological, lexical, or syntactic.

   1. Nouns are easily transferred from one language to another, but structure or function words are less easily transferred.

2. In languages that have similar syntagmatic patterns, ease of transference is, in order: verbs, adjectives, adverbs, prepositions, and interjections, which are transferred in decreasing scale.

3. Pronouns and articles show the greatest resistance to transfer.

4. The semantics of the terms used may differ from those monolinguals would assign to the same terms.

5. Transference of linguistic features may be seen from the weaker to the stronger language and vice versa.

C. Loan Words, or Borrowing, Integration

The transition from multilingualism to monolingualism in the dominant language often begins with borrowing. Language communities will borrow vocabulary from English because of its prestige, but, sometimes, because the term is nonexistent in the home language. Transfer is the preferred term rather than borrowing. Integration is the acceptance of the transferred vocabulary by the community in its everyday communications. These transfers have an impact on the vocabulary development of bilinguals who are in bilingual communities. Different types of transferred vocabulary include:

1. Loan word with no morphemic substitution, such as "taco" and "patio."

2. Hybrid or loanblends import part of the phonemic shape of the transfer such as "watchando" (watching).

3. Loanshift of loan translations do not import morphemic substitutions, such as "rascacielos" for skyscraper.

4. Loanshift is a semantic displacement, with a native term applied to a novel cultural phenomenon, such as "groceria" for grocery store.

D. Language Loss

A child's competence in the first language diminishes, while skills in the second language are not at the same level of native speakers (Schiff-Myers, 1992). The following are variables that influence the retention of a language (Conklin & Lourie, 1983). See Table 3–1 for other variables to language loss.

Table 3-1. Language Loss Patterns

Form
- Loss among forms and structures is variable
- Greater number of plural over gender errors
- Inconsistent use of morphological forms and syntactic structures
- Change in verb usage under influence of L2
- Change in verb usage is more likely to occur in cases where L1 and L2 are phonetically similar
- Stylistic shrinkage: loss of one of two "same meaning" structures
- Regular morphological alternations are reduced
- Reliance on less flexible word order
- Preference for coordinated rather than embedded constructions
- Regular morphological alternations are reduced
- Irregular patterns become regularized
- Syntactic structure of L2 is used in instances where it would be ungrammatical in L1
- Syntax used by the individual experiencing language loss is different from developmental forms used by peers

Content
- Use of L2 words for L1 words
- Inconsistent use of vocabulary in L1
- Not all lexical information is equally susceptible to loss
- Meaning extensions
- Loan translation: an idiomatic expression from the L2 is transferred to L1 where it is ungrammatical

Use
- Loss among individuals is variable
- The individual shows signs of insecurity in language performance
- The influence of L2 is most prevalent in the causal language styles of L1
- L1 loss occurs in causal language styles before formal language styles
- The amount of attention paid to speech significantly governs the outcome in L1 and L2 situations
- Language loss follows the reverse developmental pattern of second language acquisition
- The individual is aware of the language loss or weakness
- Compensatory strategies used by children are also used by adults
- Compensatory strategies used during language loss are not language bound, but they may be culturally bound
- Time elapsed since emigration only becomes relevant to language loss when there is not much contact with the native language
- Compensatory strategies used during the progression of language loss are also used during second language acquisition

---

Sources: Adapted from R.T. Anderson (1997); Altenberg (1991); Dressler (1991); Kaufman and Aranoff (1991); Maher (1991); Major (1992); Silva-Corvalan (1991); and Turian and Altenberg (1991).

1. **Political, social, and demographic factors include**

   a. Number of speakers living in concentration

   b. Recent arrival and/or continuing immigration

   c. Geographical proximity and ease of travel to native homeland

   d. High rate of return and intention to return to homeland

   e. Vocational concentration, that is employment where workers share the same language background

   f. Low social and economic mobility in mainstream occupations, and

   g. Racism and ethnic discrimination that isolates the community

2. **Cultural factors include**

   a. Native language institutions, such as churches and clubs

   b. Rel   nies requiring the language

   c. Etl   ) the language

   d. Eı   native language

   e. E   community network

   f. I   ıhance awareness of ethnic heritage

   g. Cuıtuıc .....   merican society

3. **Linguistic factors include**

   a. Use of Latin alphabet in native language makes literacy reproduction inexpensive

   b. Literacy in native language used for exchange within community

   c. Native language has international status

d. Some tolerance for loan words

E. Code Switching

Code switching is the alternating use of two languages at the word, phrase, and sentence level and when there is a complete break between languages in phonology (Valdes-Fallis, 1978).

1. Mexican children produce different kinds of code switching, depending on their age (McClure, 1977).

   a. Child code switching begins early in children and is different from adult code switching.

   b. Young children tend to mix codes by inserting single items from one language into the other. Usually English nouns, followed by adjectives, have the higher frequency of mixing into Spanish utterances, for example, "Quiero comer un hot dog" ("I want to eat a hot dog") or "Me gusta la red pelota" ("I like the red ball").

   c. At 3 years of age, code switching is used to resolve ambiguities, clarify statements, and attract attention, for example, "Mira aqui, look here."

   d. At 6 years, mode shifting, such as moving from narration to commentary, is seen through code switching.

   e. At 8 years, code switching is used for emphasis, commands, and elaboration, for example, when speaking during an English dialogue the child emphasizes by using negation in Spanish: "Te dije que no" ("I told you no").

   f. At 9 years of age, code switching may occur at the phrase and sentence level, such as, "give me the pencil que tiene un arco" ("that has a rainbow").

2. Children generally chose the language that the listeners spoke best was found by Genishi (1981).

   a. If the addressee was English dominant or monolingual, the children would use English only.

    b. If the addressee was Spanish dominant or monolingual, the children chose to use Spanish only.

3. A child who used both languages for questioning, informing, persuading, controlling, playing with language, initiating and maintaining social interaction, and personal self-expression was reported by Hudelson (1983).

4. Children learn that the rule "follow the leader" was stated by Zentella (1981).

5. Monolingual Spanish-speaking children who are in a monolingual English classroom normally remain silent in the classroom unless forced to speak was suggested by Valdes-Fallis (1978). Such children may begin to speak in English, but switch languages as an emergency attempt to continue communication.

4. There are a number of functions or use for code switching. Table 3–2 lists the reported uses of code switching among bilinguals.

7. Children should be placed among other code switching persons or a community for this ability to develop.

F. Anomie

A feeling of personal disorientation, anxiety, and social isolation (Baetens-Beardsmore, 1986).

1. Child (1943) observed symptoms of frustration in the children of Italian immigrants in New York.

    a. These children experienced conflicts of loyalties between the home language and the dominant culture.

    b. Child (1943) reported that, for these children, the conflict was resolved by withdrawing either from the outside culture or from the home language and culture. The latter brought about feelings of turmoil and severance from the family.

2. Baetens-Beardsmore (1986) states that this situation becomes more acute for the adolescent who is trying to develop a set of personality traits in two languages.

Table 3–2. Stylistic Code Switching

Function	Description
Quotation	Code switch marks a direct quotation
Repetition	Message in one code is repeated in the second code
Addressee specification	Code switch singles out one of several possible interlocutors
Clarification	Code switch functions to resolve ambiguity or clarify a potential or apparent lack of understanding
Emphasis	Message is emphatically underscored in the second code
Elaboration	Code switch adds additional information to original message
Personalization	Code contrast reflects personal opinion versus known fact
Interjection	Code switch serves to mark an interjection or filler
Topic shift	Code contrast used to mark a desired change in topic
Preformulation	Code contrast marks automatic speech and linguistic routines
Paraphrase	Message in one code is paraphrased in the second code

Source: From "Considerations in the Assessment and Treatment of Neurogenic Disorders in Bilingual Adults," by B. A. Reyes. In *Bilingual Speech-Language Pathology: An Hispanic Focus* (p. 166), by H. Kayser (Ed.), 1995, San Diego: Singular Publishing Group, Inc., Copyright 1995 by Singular Publishing Group, Inc. Reprinted with permission.

2. McCloskey and Schaar (1965) have suggested that anomie may be highest among persons of low education, low income, and low prestige occupations. As the individual learns more about the second language, its cultural values and norms, the standard that is expected from the second language learner becomes higher.

V. FRAMEWORKS FOR EXAMINING LANGUAGE DEVELOPMENT IN BILINGUALS

Note: This section provides frameworks and milestones of bilingualism for speech-language pathologists to use in their assessment and intervention programs with bilingual children. (See also Appendixes A and

B.) There are other excellent resources beyond this volume that provide literature reviews about infant and adult second-language acquisition.

Kessler (1984), McLaughlin (1984), and Grosjean (1982) describe three groups of children who are exposed to two languages in childhood. These include simultaneous bilingual, preschool successive bilingual, and school-age successive bilingual children. They are described in terms of when the second language is introduced into the child's environment.

A. Simultaneous Bilingual

A term for children who learn two languages in the home before the age of 3 years. Either:

1. A child has bilingual parents or

2. Parents speak different languages, that is, mixed-language families.

B. The Preschool Successive Bilingual

A child who learns the second language after 3 years of age, who is either:

1. A child who enters a preschool program to learn a minority language for enrichment or

2. A Spanish-speaking child who enters a Head Start program.

C. The School-age Successive Bilingual

A term for children who learn a second language after beginning school at age 5 or 6 years.

VI. COMMUNICATIVE COMPETENCY

Kessler (1984) describes bilingualism in children in terms of the communicative competency they must achieve in both languages. The child must learn the grammatical, sociolinguistic, discourse, and strategic competencies necessary to communicate successfully in their group or community.

A. Grammatical or linguistic competence is the mastery of phonological, syntactic, and lexical features of the language.

B. Sociolinguistic competence addresses the sociocultural rules of appropriate language use. This involves knowledge of the rules for who, what, how, and when to speak with members of the community who have varying status and roles.

C. Discourse competence involves the connection of utterances to form a meaningful entity, for example, in narratives and conversations. Once a child is in a school setting, the discourse rules become more complex, with the addition of rules for lectures, book reviews, and other discourse events.

D. Strategic competence involves strategies that are drawn on to compensate for breakdowns in communication when there is imperfect knowledge of the rules in the other areas of communicative competence.

   1. These strategies include paraphrasing, repetitions, circumlocutions, message modifications, hesitations, and avoidance of difficult words, phrases, or situations.

   2. Strategic competency is an important ability in second language acquisition.

VII. SIMULTANEOUS BILINGUALISM (BIRTH TO 3 YEARS).

A. The research concerning typical children at this age appears to support several conclusions:

   1. These children do not have any difficulties in comprehension and may have only one lexical system in the initial development of their vocabulary (Volterra & Taeschner, 1978).

   2. There does not appear to be any difference between these youngsters and monolinguals when comparing milestones in language development, such as when first words, number of words, and word combinations appear.

   3. These children's linguistic context and interactions are important in the acquisition of the two languages. That is, who is using the language and how much exposure the child is receiving for each language are both important for the potential bilingualism of the child.

B. There appears to be disagreement among the research data in areas of lexical and phonological interference and linguistic production.

1. Lexical interference exists from the beginning of first words.

2. Children may or may not have phonological interference, that is, some children use the phonological systems to distinguish the two languages and separate the languages by the sound system.

3. Children's linguistic production also varies with bilingual homes. Some children reared in balanced bilingual homes may become bilingual and others may not.

C. Three stages in the bilingual development of three English-Italian-speaking children were observed by Volterra and Taeschner (1978).

1. In stage 1, the children had only one lexical system, which included words from both languages. These children had words in English that did not have equivalents in Italian and vice versa. Both languages were used indiscriminately, as one would use one language.

2. In stage 2, the children differentiated the two lexical systems, but used only one grammar. They were relating the lexical items in a manner more like semantic relationships.

3. Stage 3 was a complete separation of the lexical and grammar systems. The children used each language without mixing. Leopold (1949) and Fantini (1978) reported that this stage occurred between 3 and 3.6 years of age. This observation is important because **many Hispanic preschoolers enter the schools with a mixture of the two languages** and have not yet separated the two systems. Some children may need additional time to learn to differentiate the two languages.

D. Leopold (1949) studied his daughter Hildegard's development of English and German. She heard English from her mother and German from her father.

1. Hildegard had an initial mixed language stage but

2. Slowly separated the two languages systems

3. Had accompanying awareness of her bilingualism.

4. Leopold noted that there was an immediate influence on one language system when the linguistic environment favored that language.

5. There was also avoidance of difficult words and constructions in the weaker language, German.

6. His final observation was that there was complete separation of the phonological and grammar systems, but there was an enduring influence of the dominant language on the other in the area of vocabulary and idioms.

7. He stated that Hildegard had balanced bilingual abilities by the time she was 5 years of age. Hildegard did have a preference in languages, and we must be aware that children at young ages do become attached or may favor one language over the other.

E. Fantini (1978) provided a sociolinguistic perspective on the simultaneous bilingualism of his son, Mario. He found that children at a young age have influence on how two languages are learned and which language will be preferred.

1. Age 1.4, first words in Spanish

2. Age 1.8–1.10, discriminates between languages. Fantini described Mario as affectionate and friendly to persons who spoke in Spanish. But when individuals used English, Mario was distant and would not talk to the speaker.

3. Age 2.6, first words in English

4. Age 2.7–2.8, mixed English and Spanish

5. Age 2.8, classifies speakers by appearance. Mario learned that Hispanics had a certain appearance and that places such as Mexico, Venezuela, and South Texas were areas where Spanish was primarily spoken.

6. Age 3.0–3.4, differentiated language use by persons

7. Age 3.4, differentiated language use by place.

8. Age 3.6, used term *Español* and age 3.9, used term *English.*

9. Age 4.1, asked for translations.

10. Age 4.2, tells others what languages he speaks.

11. Age 5.4, teacher reported a problem in conversational rules.

12. Age 5.8, recognized accents.

13. Age 7.5, could recognize proficiency level in Spanish

14. Age 7.11–8.1, recognized regional dialects of English and Spanish

15. Age 8.2, used code switching to exclude individuals from conversations.

16. Mario's use differed with adults, sibling, and peers; including intimacy, peer talk, baby talk, and an adult style.

F. Narratives

Heath (1986) states that every society allows its young to hear and produce at least four basic narrative genres.

1. Recounts
Adults ask children to relate a shared experience to another person. Recounts are rarely heard in the Mexican-American community.

2. Event Casts
The individual describes an activity that is occurring at the moment or is planned for the future. Among Mexican Americans, these never occur in daily events, but occur when the family cooperatively plans for future events.

3. Accounts
The teller provides information that is unknown to the listener or offers further explanations of what the listener already knows. This is most common type of genre among Mexican-American communities.

4. Stories

The individual describes an animate being who moves through a series of events with goal-directed behavior. Stories told are about both family members and historical figures.

G. Strategic Competency

Children have a variety of strategies to help them learn language.

1. **Gestalt Versus Analytical** (Peters-Mink, 1977)
   Some children must approach language learning by looking at whole units or events, while other children must break down the units into smaller sections to determine meaning and rules.

2. **Metalinguistic Strategies** (Snyder-McLean & McLean, 1978)
   Children may determine the rules by thinking about the regular patterns in the language that is spoken.

3. **Learning Versus Cognitive Strategies** (Corder, 1967)
   Communicative strategies are used to communicate effectively, while learning strategies are mental processes to help construct the rules of the language.

4. Wong-Fillmore (1979) describes cognitive and social strategies that are similar to Corder's communicative and learning strategies. Social strategies include joining groups and acting as if you understand, using choice words to give the impression of expressive abilities in the language, and counting on friends for help when a topic is not understood. Cognitive strategies include the assumption that speech is related to the context, guessing, analysis of repeated phrases, and focusing on the big picture rather than the finer parts of the language.

5. Chesterfield and Chesterfield (1985) state that older children use a number of other strategies, such as imitation, deferred practice, asking informants, reading, observation, using a dictionary, silent practice, asking for repetition, and many others.

VIII. RESEARCH METHODOLOGY

Research in second-language acquisition and speech-language impairments is appearing in professional journals. Reviewing this emerging literature requires a critical eye by the speech-language pathologist. Following are

McLaughlin's (1984a) recommendations for reviewing the literature and determining the investigation's validity.

A. **Look for bias** in any form in the design of the study.

B. **Critique the hypothesis** for conflict with previous research

C. Review and Critique

1. Number, gender, and ages of the subjects.

2. Socioeconomic status of the subjects.

3. Educational background of families and subjects.

4. Intelligence levels.

5. Description of bilingualism in the subjects.

6. Length of residence and exposure to English.

7. Proficiency levels in each language by subjects.

8. Description of

   a. measure(s), including reliability and validity.

   b. mixing and code-switching events.

9. Attitude of subjects and family toward bilingualism.

C H A P T E R

4

Nonbiased Assessment

In assessment, the evaluator must be sensitive to potential cultural biases of a test, possess the ability to be flexible in testing, and have the knowledge to derive sufficient information from nonstandardized testing to make professional judgments about a child's language capabilities. Once a child is targeted for formal testing, the speech-language pathologist must be cautious in selecting appropriate assessment tools. The most common forms of test bias that arise in assessment of culturally and linguistically diverse (CLD) children are: (1) The child's cultural group is inadequately represented in the normative sample, (2) The child has limited familiarity with or uses a variation of the language of the test, (3) The child is unfamiliar with situations presented in the test stimuli, and (4) The child holds different values from those presented in the test.

Test instruments are used to determine if there is a speech and/or language impairment and to describe the performance of an individual on a task. When no instruments are available for the Spanish speaker, or the instruments used are translated from English versions, or the clinician must prepare criterion-referenced instruments, the instruments fall below the high standards for assessment we provide to English speakers.

This chapter reviews the procedures recommended for speech-language pathology and special education in assessing communicative impairments in Hispanic children. A discussion follows about prereferrals, and includes case histories, questionnaires, and observations. Test instruments, their use, and how they can be adapted to fit the needs of students are briefly discussed. Modified procedures, including a brief discussion of dynamic assessment, are also presented. Assessment checklists and the interpretation of data are briefly presented. The chapter concludes with other important considerations in the assessment process.

I. REFERRAL CHARACTERISTICS

The child is initially reviewed by a school child study team whose purpose is to help teachers determine the difficulties that children have in the classroom. Child study teams should be gatekeepers for special education, but they often function more as processors to only enroll students into special education (Garcia & Ortiz, 1988). Reynolds (1984) reported that 75 to 90% of students who are referred to child study teams are placed in special education.

A. Kayser (1985) described clinicians as having perceived eight demographic characteristics as being common to the Mexican-American children labeled having language impairment and placed in their caseloads. These could easily identify any second-language learner as having communication impairment and included:

1. Low socioeconomic level;

2. Monolingual Spanish-speaking parents;

3. English-only speaking teachers and classrooms;

4. Academic difficulties, primarily in reading;

5. Comprehension difficulties;

6. Referral in the second through fourth grades;

7. Poor conversational skills; and

8. Being bilingual or predominantly English speaking.

B. **The prereferral process is necessary** to avoid overreferral to special education and the possibility of inappropriate identification of Hispanic children as having communication impairment.

II. OTHER CHARACTERISTICS

Bilingual children with speech and language impairments have other characteristics described in the literature (Ambert, 1986a, 1986b; Damico, Oller, & Storey 1983; Kayser, 1990; Langdon, 1983; Linares-Orama & Sanders, 1977; Maldonado, 1984; Merino, 1983; Taylor, 1986), including:

A. Receptive Language

The children lack the ability to:

1. Associate sounds with objects or experiences

2. Discriminate tones, phonemes, and morphemes

3. Remember words

4. Understand who, what, where, and why questions

B. Expressive Language

The children lack the ability to:

1. Produce phonemes /s/, /l/, /r/, and /rr/. The child may substitute, omit, and distort sounds; reverse the order of sounds in words; or coalesce or shorten words. (See Appendix C for a Test of Oral and Verbal Apraxia.)

2. Produce articles, pronouns, prepositions, copulas "ser" and "estar," auxilliary "estar," reflexive pronoun "se," plural endings, and conjunctions. These children use incorrect word order, substitute the schwa for articles, pronouns, and other grammatical structures. The child may have difficulty with noun-verb and article-noun agreement and confuse verb tenses.

3. There may be inappropriate verbal labels for common objects, actions, and persons. Circumlocutions may be used when the child cannot retrieve specific words. There may be difficulty with retelling stories or narrating personal experiences, classifying events

with verbal labels, and organizing words in appropriate sentences. There may be an inability to correct grammatical errors in sentence constructions and difficulty with problem solving.

4. Friendships may be limited to low achievers, indiscrete gestures are used with friends, and there are limited group interactions with classmates. The child has fewer strategies than other children to seek clarification. The child does not organize games among peers or have conversations with them. His or her communication has little or no effect on the actions of peers.

C. **A number of language and attention behaviors,** listed by Ortiz and Maldonado-Colón (1986), are used by special educators to identify students with learning disability students. According to Ortiz and Maldonado-Colón, these same behaviors may also be observed in second language learners. These include:

1. Short attention span,

2. Distractability,

3. Daydreams,

4. Demands immediate gratification,

5. Disorganized,

6. Unable to stay on task, and

7. Appears confused.

D. **Descriptions of the language behaviors common** to both second language learners and students with learning disability (Ortiz & Maldonado-Colon, 1986) include:

1. Speaks infrequently,

2. Uses gestures,

3. Speaks in single words or phrases,

4. Refuses to answer questions,

5. Does not volunteer information,

6. Comments inappropriately,

7. Has poor recall,

8. Has poor comprehension,

9. Has poor vocabulary,

10. Has difficulty sequencing ideas,

11. Has difficulty sequencing events,

12. Is unable to tell or retell stories,

13. Confuses similar sounding words,

14. Has poor pronunciation, and

15. Has poor syntax.

F. **Mattes and Omark (1991) and Kayser (1990)** suggest that students with language-impairment who are bilingual have difficulty in discourse with peers. Peer relationships are valued among Hispanic students.

1. Child rarely initiates verbal interactions with peers.

2. Child rarely initiates interactions in peer group activities.

3. Child rarely initiates or organizes play activities with peers.

4. Child does not respond verbally when verbal interactions are initiated by peers.

5. Child's communication has little or no effect on the actions of peers.

6. Child does not engage in dialogue/conversations with peers.

7. Child communicates with limited number of classroom peers.

8. Child generally uses gestures rather than speech to communicate with peers.

9. Facial expressions, eye contact, and other nonverbal aspects of the child's communication are perceived by peers as inappropriate.

10. Facial expressions and/or actions of peers indicate that they may be having difficulty understanding the child's oral and/or nonverbal communications.

11. Peers rarely initiate verbal interactions with the child.

G. Roseberry-McKibbin (1995) suggests the following as possible characteristics of children who may have a language learning disability.

1. Nonverbal aspects of language are culturally inappropriate.

2. Student does not express basic needs adequately.

3. Student rarely initiates verbal interaction with peers.

4. When peers initiate interaction, student responds inappropriately.

5. Student replaces speech with gestures, communicates nonverbally when talking would be expected.

6. Peers give indications that they have difficulty understanding the student.

7. Student often gives inappropriate responses.

8. Student has difficulty conveying thoughts in an organized, sequential manner that is understandable to listeners.

9. Student shows poor topic maintenance.

10. Student has word finding difficulties that go beyond normal second language acquisition patterns.

11. Student fails to provide significant information to the listener, leaving the listener confused.

12. Student has difficulty with conversational turn-taking skills.

13. Student perseverates on a topic, even after the topic has changed.

14. Student fails to ask and answer questions appropriately.

15. Student needs to have information repeated, even when the information is stated simply and comprehensibly.

16. Student often echoes what the child hears.

III. PREREFERRAL

The purpose of prereferrals is to reduce the number of inappropriate referrals to speech-language services and special education (Ortiz & Maldonado-Colon, 1986).

A. Screening and intervention as a prereferral is described by Olson (1991) as identifying the following:

   1. Child's problems,

   2. Source of the problems, and

   3. Steps to resolve the difficulties within the classroom setting.

B. An 8-step prereferral process that will help reduce inappropriate referrals for second language learners was described by Garcia and Ortiz (1988). The basis of these steps is to modify the curriculum and teaching strategies to assist students to learn.

   1. Is the curriculum known to be effective for linguistically culturally diverse students? If no, adapt, supplement, and develop the curriculum. If yes, then proceed

   2. Is the student having academic difficulty? If no, then there is no problem and the process ends. If yes, then proceed.

   3. Is there evidence that the child did not learn what was taught? If no, then check within and between classroom settings, individuals, teacher perceptions, and student's work samples. If yes, then proceed.

4. Is there evidence of systematic efforts to identify the source of difficulty and take corrective action? If no, then look at teacher qualifications, experience, track record, teaching style, expectations, perceptions, instructional management, and behavior management skills. Also, look at the student's cultural characteristics, socioeconomic status, cognitive/learning style, modes of communication, patterns of participation, language proficiency, locus of control/attribution, self-concept, motivation, experiential background, and affective filter. If yes, then proceed.

5. Do student difficulties persist? If no, then problem solving was successful and the process ends. If yes, then proceed.

6. Have other programming alternatives been tried? If no, then determine program/placement alternatives such as bilingual education, and so on. If yes, then proceed.

7. Do difficulties continue although alternatives are tried? If no, then the student remains in the alternative program, as appropriate. If yes, then proceed.

8. Referral to special education.

C. **For the speech-language pathologist,** the goal of prereferral is to assist the special education team in determining the child's language environment (home and school), language use (home and school), and bilingual proficiency.

IV. OTHER SOURCES OF INFORMATION

To determine a child's language environment, use, and bilingual proficiency one can also explore the case history, questionnaires, and observation of the student.

A. Case History

Meitus and Weinberg (1983) suggest taking a detailed case history with 10 categories for investigation. Mexican families should be given specific questions, and adequate time must be allowed for the family to think about their responses. A personal interview and review of the information with the parent is important to ensure the completeness of the responses to all of the questions (Kayser, 1995a). The Meitus and Weinberg (1983) categories are:

1. Conditions related to the onset,

2. Conditions related to development of the problem,

3. Previous diagnostic results,

4. Previous rehabilitation results,

5. General developmental status,

6. Health status,

7. Educational/vocational status,

8. Emotional/social adjustment,

9. Pertinent family concerns, and

10. Other information volunteered by the respondent. (See Appendix D.)

11. Langdon (1992) suggests the following be included in case history information.

   a. Reason for referral.

   b. Sources of information (e.g., cumulative record, other staff's oral or written reports, parent/family personal or telephone interview).

   c. Social and family background, such as place of birth, sibling position, and number of persons living with the student.

   d. Languages spoken in the family.

   e. Parents' occupation, educational level, and proficiency in English.

   f. Language or learning difficulty of other family members.

   g. Visits to home country.

   h. Parents' perception of the student,

i. Student's experiences with literacy and activities outside of the home.

j. Health and developmental background.

k. Specific programs that the student has attended.

l. Reading programs followed and modifications made to meet the student's needs.

m. School attendance record and any disruptions in education.

n. Observations and comments of other staff members.

o. Results of other testing.

p. Observations made during school and testing event.

B. Questionnaires

Mattes and Omark (1991) and Langdon and Cheng (1992) provide lists of these instruments. Very few of these questionnaires have had the validity and reliability determined for the questions. Speech-language pathologists should follow up all questions on a questionnaire with additional probing and specific questions to ensure that parent respondents understand the questions and that correct information is conveyed to the clinician.

C. Observations

Observations of children should be documented in a systematic manner using the previously listed characteristics as guidelines for the observation. Omark (1981) described two observational techniques that may be used to document student behaviors: scan and focal techniques (see Tables 4–1 & 4–2).

1. **Scan technique.** The speech-language pathologist observes specific behaviors during normal interactions among a group of children in a classroom.

    a. The observer notes the activity of one child for 10 to 20 minutes, taking a frequency count of specific behaviors.

Table 4–1. Observable Communicative Behaviors for Spanish- and English-Speaking Students with Language Impairment

1. Child rarely initiates verbal interactions with peers.
2. Child rarely initiates interactions in peer group activities.
3. Child rarely initiates or organizes play activities with peers.
4. Child does not respond verbally when verbal interactions are initiated by peers.
5. Child's communication has little or no effect on the actions of peers.
6. Child does not engage in dialogue/conversations with peers.
7. Child communicates with limited number of classroom peers.
8. Child generally uses gestures rather than speech to communicate with peers.
9. Facial expressions, eye contact, and other nonverbal aspects of the child's communication are perceived by peers as inappropriate.
10. Facial expressions and/or actions of peers indicate that they may be having difficulty understanding the child's oral and/or nonverbal communications.
11. Peers rarely initiate verbal interactions with the child.

Source: From "Assessment of Speech and Language Impairments in Bilingual Children," by H. Kayser, In *Bilingual Speech Language Pathology: An Hispanic Focus* (p. 250), by H. Kayser (Ed.), 1995, San Diego: Singular Publishing Group, Inc. Copyright 1995 by Singular Publishing Group Inc. Reprinted with permission.

> **b.** The observer then moves to the second and third child and observes the same behaviors for the same length of time.
>
> **c.** This information may be tallied and compared to past and/or future observations of the target student and peers.

2. **Focal technique.** This technique concentrates on the behaviors of one student over an extended time.

> **a.** The observer notes the child's language behaviors for a number of days or weeks.
>
> **b.** The sampling is accumulative and compared over time for the same child.
>
> **c.** The procedure provides more information than what would be observed in the scan technique.

V. SPEECH AND LANGUAGE ASSESSMENT INSTRUMENTS

Mattes and Omark (1991) and Langdon and Cheng (1992) list the available Spanish tests published in the United States. The majority of the tests are

Table 4–2. Student Behavior Checklist

Attention/Order	Personal/Emotional	Interpersonal/Social	Adult Relations/Authority	School Adaptation	Language
*Short attention span	Sad/unhappy	Has few friends	Talks back to adults	Disrupts other students	Speaks excessively
*Distractible	*Nervous/anxious	Verbally aggressive	Intimidated by authority	Speaks out of turn	*Speaks infrequently
Talks excessively	*Shy/timid	**Denies responsibility for actions	Overly anxious to please	**Does not complete assignments	*Uses gestures
*Daydreams	Short tempered	Instigates misbehaviors in others	**Passive/uncooperative	**Cannot work independently	*Speaks in single words or phrases
Unable to wait turn	*Poor self-confidence	*Easily influenced	Distrustful of adults	Copies other's work	*Refuses to answer Questions
Loud and noisy	Extreme mood changes	Bossy	Refuses to accept limits	**Exerts little effort	*Does not volunteer information
Constant need for stimulation	Cries easily	**Demands attention	**Defiant	**Lacks interest/apathetic	*Comments inappropriately
Hyperactive	Unusual mannerisms or habits	Inconsiderate	Ambivalent toward adults	Frequently tardy or absent	*Poor recall
*Demands immediate gratification	*Fearful	Selfish	Uses profanity	**Gives up easily	*Poor comprehension
*Disorganized	Easily excitable	Lies	**Clings to adults	**Cannot manage time	*Poor vocabulary
*Unable to stay on task	Inappropriate emotional responses	Steals	**Overly dependent	**Lacks drive	*Difficulty sequencing ideas
	Immature	Jealous	**Seeks constant praise	**Disorganized	*Difficulty sequencing events
	Toileting problems	Can't keep hands to self	Rebellious	**Cannot plan	*Unable to tell or retell stories
	*Difficulty in adjusting to new situations	Manipulates others	**Needs teacher direction and feedback	**Unable to tolerate change	*Confuses similar Sounding words
	Cruel	Suspicious		**Sporadic academic performances	*Poor pronunciation
	Uncooperative	*Cannot handle criticism		Makes excuses	*Poor syntax/grammar
	Loses control	**Avoids competition		Destructive	
	Overacts	Prefers to be alone		**Does not initiate	
		Physically aggressive		Needs reminding	

*Normal behavior characteristics—often referred because different from expectations.

**Behavior characteristics frequently associated with learning disabilities.

Source: From *Bilingualism and Learning Disabilities: Policy and Practice for Teachers and Administrators* (pp. 40—41). Edited by A. C. Willig and H. F. Greenberg, 1986, New York, American Library Publishing Co. Copyright 1986, by American Library Publishing Co., P.O. Box 4272, Sedona, AZ 86340. Reprinted with permission.

described as having poor reliability and validity. Table 4–3 summarizes criticisms of the use of standardized tests with culturally and linguistically diverse populations. Appendix F lists publishers, tests, and materials for Spanish speakers.

A. Adapting Tests

Adapting a test instrument means that the tasks and content of the instrument are changed to include culturally appropriate stimuli (Gavillan-Torres,1984; Kayser, 1989) and are therefore less biased for the culturally and linguistically diverse child.

1. Kayser (1989) suggests that a team of bilingual professionals develop the adapted test instrument.

2. Appendix E is a screening test developed for Head Start children and then adapted for Mexican-American preschoolers.

B. Questions and strategies for use by bilingual professionals to adapt test instruments were reviewed by Kayser (1989).

1. Questions

a. What is it measuring?

b. Is knowledge typical of home, school, academic, preschool settings?

c. What type of experiences are necessary to "pass" a subtest?

d. Do tasks appear to be "unnatural" for Hispanic members of a review committee?

e. Can the members of the review committee perform the tasks?

f. Appropriateness for which age/grade levels?

2. Strategies

a. Divide task into receptive and expressive modes.

b. Discuss how task could be changed to tap a similar skill/ability.

Table 4–3. Test Criticism Checklist

1. Lack of validity (Does not measure what it is intended to measure). The test does not have:
   a. **Face validity** (appearance of soundness)
   b. **Content validity** (representativeness of tasks on tests with larger sample of behavior)
   c. **Predictive validity** (prediction of some later success)
   d. **Concurrent validity** (results given that are similar to existing tests)
   e. **Construct validity** (a valid theory of nature of language and language learning reflected)
2. Lack of reliability (does not consistently give same results). The test does not have:
   a. **Split-half correlations**
   b. **Parallel forms**
   c. **Retesting using the same test**
   d. **Explicit ratings criteria**
3. Standardization and norms do not include the group to be tested.
4. Development of test construction is limited.
5. Content of tests are biased by:
   a. **Author(s) of test**
   b. **Standardization group**
   c. **Dialect and language group**
   d. **Difficulty of items**
6. Tests are biased by:
   a. **Use of middle-class mainstream values and experiences**
   b. **Not reflecting other cultural groups' experiences**
7. Tests foster low expectancy for culturally and linguistically diverse children.
8. Tests shape curriculum and do not lead to meaningful instruction.
9. Tests evaluate only a segment of a child's communicative abilities.
10. Tests are viewed as accurate and fixed assessments of a child's communicative abilities.
11. Tests are not purely objective.
12. Tests lack linguistic realism and authenticity.

Source: From "Assessment of Speech and Language Impairments in Bilingual Children," by H. Kayser. In *Bilingual Speech-Language Pathology: An Hispanic Focus* (p. 251), by H. Kayser (Ed.), 1995, San Diego: Singular Publishing Group, Inc. Copyright 1995 by Singular Publishing Group Inc. Reprinted with permission.

   c. Share professionals' experiences in administering particular subtests to Hispanic children.

   d. Review past folders for success/failure with a subtest in question.

   e. Determine appropriateness of vocabulary for community and children.

f. Determine developmental sequence in vocabulary through review with experiences of teachers and community members.

g. Solicit committee reactions to picture stimuli for accuracy of picture representations.

h. Develop story content that is familiar for the subject area with topics, objects, and animals that are found within the community.

C. Procedure Modification

Modifying procedures requires a clinician to change personal standardized procedures to those that best elicit a child's responses. There are three phases for implementing modified procedures: before, during, and after testing (Erickson & Iglesias, 1986; Kayser, 1989).

1. Before Testing
Preliminary precautions should be taken in the period just before the testing session begins and these should be documented for future testing to include the same procedures. The process requires preparation time but is considered to be effective.

a. Reword the instructions so that phrasing, terms, and sentence structure are familiar to the child to assist the youngster in understanding test materials and what is expected of him or her.

b. Develop additional practice items to offer the child more examples of the test stimuli.

c. Obtain and use different picture stimuli that may be more representative of the child's culture or provide better examples of the item.

d. Omit items that you know from your experience are incorrectly identified by Hispanic children.

2. During Testing
The following modified procedures are presented from the easiest to implement to the most difficult, that is, in ascending order of difficulty.

a. Record all responses, especially if the child changes an answer.

b. Repeat the test stimuli when necessary and more frequently than what is specified or allowed in the test manual.

c. Provide additional time for the child to respond.

d. Watch the child's eye gaze and body movements for referencing when there is no verbal response.

e. Accept culturally appropriate responses as correct.

f. On vocabulary recognition tests, have the child name the picture in addition to pointing to the stimulus item to ascertain the appropriateness of the label for the pictorial representation.

g. Have the child identify the actual object, body part, action, photograph, and so forth, particularly if he or she has limited experience with books, line drawings, or the testing process.

h. Have the child explain why an "incorrect" answer was selected.

i. Continue testing beyond the ceiling of the test.

3. After Testing

a. Compare the child's responses to charts on dialect and/or second-language acquisition features.

b. Rescore articulation and expressive language samples, giving credit for variation or differences.

c. If the child was uncooperative or unresponsive, complete the testing in several sessions.

d. Consider having a peer, sibling, parent, or trusted adult administer the test items during a second session.

D. Using Norm-referenced Tests with Culturally and Linguistically Diverse Populations

Two problems may arise in using norm referenced tests (Lopez, Cheng, & Kayser (1995):

1. Overinterpreting the scores obtained on the test.

    a. Norms are scores derived from a representative sampling of the performance by a large group of subjects and the individual is compared to the group.

    b. The norms on the test tell you how normal children perform on specific language tasks when the test is administered in a specified manner.

    c. The norms are not used if the test was administered in a nonstandardized format.

  2. Norms do not equate to ability and developmental sequence.

    a. Norms do not provide precise measurements of the ability of every child.

    b. Norms do not imply a developmental sequence of behaviors.

VI. TEST ADMINISTRATION

There are variables that must be considered as part of actual testing. The following are questions that should be considered to determine if the assessment of the child is valid (Lopez, Cheng, & Kayser, 1995).

A. Testing Procedures

A number of practices may be used by speech-language pathologists in testing bilingual Hispanic children. Evaluating Hispanic children requires more time and effort than testing an English monolingual student. Using questionable and abbreviated methods for Hispanic students results in invalid assessment results.

  1. The translation of tests. Directly translating a test does not necessarily equate to an appropriately adapted assessment instrument (Erickson & Iglesias, 1986; Kayser, 1989). If a test is translated, it should be developed by a team of bilingual professionals. The reasons for the difficulty of translating tests rests on how languages differ in a number of areas:

    a. Honorifics (formal *used* versus familiar *tu*). Some languages have two or more informal and formal forms to address individuals.

b. **Gender markers** (*el* and *la*). Gender must be marked in two or more words in one utterance.

c. **Semantics** (*arroz*, tomato-based and spicy for Spanish connotation versus *rice*, being white or brown for Anglos); What is translated may connote a different meaning in the second language.

d. **Structural rules** (adjective before noun versus adjective after noun); The word order may vary between the languages.

e. **Registers** (formal educated versus *barrio*); a translated form may stigmatize social class differences.

f. **Dialectal variations** in vocabulary and registers (Cuban versus Mexican); There are differences in semantics and pragmatics for different Hispanic groups.

g. **Cultural norms** for who speaks what to whom and when. What is translated may be inappropriate for an Hispanic child to say or respond to in their culture.

2. **Clinician language proficiency.** There are two issues relative to the assessment of Spanish-speaking children that may have a biasing effect on the child's test performance: the clinician's Spanish or English language proficiency and dialect.

a. **Dialect.** The dialect may have an effect on children's comprehension, especially if the child has speech and language impairment. Allowing a child to listen to the clinician's speech patterns during a 10-minute conversational period may improve the child's performance on tests. The same may be true if the child's dialect uses a slower rate of speech than what the clinician uses in her or his dialect.

b. **The clinician's language proficiency.** A clinician's limited proficiency or lack of native-like use of the language may have potential effects on a child's performance on test instruments. This should be considered and monitored for potential biasing effects on children's test performance.

c. **American Speech-Language-Hearing Association's (ASHA) bilingual clinician definition.** "Speech-language pathologists or audiologists who present themselves as bilingual for the purposes of providing clinical services must be able to speak their primary language and to speak (or sign) at least one other language with native or near-native proficiency in lexicon (vocabulary), semantics (meaning), phonology (pronunciation), morphology/syntax (grammar), and pragmatics (uses) during clinical management. To provide bilingual assessment and remediation services in the client's language, the bilingual speech-language pathologist or audiologist (Asha, 1989) should possess:

(1) Ability to describe the process of normal speech and language acquisition for both bilingual and monolingual individuals and how those processes are manifested in oral (or manually coded) and written language;

(2) Ability to administer and interpret formal and informal assessment procedures to distinguish between communication differences and communication disorders in oral (or manually coded) and written language;

(3) Ability to apply intervention strategies for treatment of communicative disorders in a client's native language; and

(4) Ability to recognize cultural factors which affect the delivery of speech-language pathology and audiology services to the client's language community."

B. Questions

1. Are there factors (attitude, physical conditions) supporting the need to reschedule this child for evaluation at another time?

2. Could the physical environment of this test setting adversely affect this child's performance (e.g., room temperature, poor lighting, noise, furnishings inappropriate for the child's size, and space inadequacy)?

3. Am I familiar with the test manual and have I followed its directions?

4. Have I given this child clear directions?

5. If his or her native language is not English, have I instructed the youngster in his or her language?

6. Am I sure that this child understands my directions?

7. Have I accurately recorded entire responses to test items so that I might later consider them when interpreting his or her test scores items, even though the child's answers may be incorrect?

8. Did I establish and maintain rapport with this child throughout the evaluation session?

9. Has the stronger language been tested and have both languages been tested?

VII. SCORING AND INTERPRETATION

Observing the child's performance on the test items after the testing is an excellent indicator of the validity of the responses obtained (Lopez, Cheng, & Kayser, 1995). Questions to ask are:

A. **Have I examined** each item missed by this child, rather than merely looking at the total score?

B. **Is there a pattern** to the types of items this child missed?

C. **Are the items missed** free of cultural bias?

D. **If I omitted all items missed that are culturally biased,** would this child have performed significantly better?

E. **Am I aware that I must** consider other factors in the interpretation of this child's scores?

F. **Have I considered** the effect the child's attitude and/or physical condition may have had on his or her performance?

G. **Have I considered** the effect that the child's possible lack of rapport with me may have had on his or her performance?

H. **Have I reported and interpreted** scores within a range rather than as a number?

I. **Will I allow test scores to outweigh** my professional judgment about this child?

VIII. EXAMINING COLLECTED DATA (Kayser, 1995a) CHECKLIST

A. **Identify parental or client** concerns that have been met.

B. **Identify possible neurogenic** etiology.

C. **Observe sequencing,** memory, and attention span results.

D. **Consider the possibility** of language loss.

E. **Observe the variety** of forms, use, and content in different contexts.

F. **Observe code switching** and language mixing in the language samples.

G. **Observe whether** the specific speech and language problems exist in both languages.

IX. CONSULTATION WITH TRANSDISCIPLINARY TEAM MEMBERS AND OTHERS

A. **Have I met with the team** to share my findings regarding this child?

B. **Are other team members' evaluation results** in conflict with mine?

C. **Can I admit my discipline's limitations** and seek assistance from other team members?

D. **Do I willingly share my competencies** and knowledge with other team members for the benefit of this child?

E. **Has the team arrived at its conclusions** as a result of team consensus, or was our decision influenced by the personality and/or power of an individual team member?

X. ASSESSMENT REPORT

The report is the most important product of the evaluation, because it will convey to the parents and other professionals the results of the speech-language pathologist's expert analysis of a child's strengths and weaknesses. The following are questions to answer in writing the report (Kayser, 1995a; Langdon, 1992).

A. **Is my report clearly written** and free of jargon, so that it can be easily understood by this child, his or her parents, and teachers?

B. **Does my report answer** the questions posed in the referral?

C. **Are the recommendations** I have made realistic and practical for the child, school, teacher, and parents?

D. **Have I provided** alternative recommendations?

E. **Have I included** in my report a description of any unusual circumstances or difficulties that I encountered and the effects of these problems during the assessment process?

F. **Have I reported** any test adaptations?

G. **Have I reported** the nature of the evaluation, for example, use of an interpreter?

XI. ALTERNATIVE ASSESSMENTS: PORTFOLIO AND DYNAMIC

A. Portfolio Assessment

Portfolio/authentic assessment is a collection of student work samples that reflects the student's achievements, growth, and efforts in one or more selected areas (e.g., reading, writing, listening, speaking). It measures a child's performance on meaningful tasks that are relevant to classroom learning and real-world activities. Children and teachers establish evaluation parameters for portfolios. One primary advantage of the portfolio is that, instead of emphasizing what the child cannot do, it provides an opportunity for the child to show what he or she can do without time constraints. M. Gottlieb provides portfolio assessment advantages (personal communication, February 6, 1998):

1. Presents students' authentic work as evidence.

2. Shows students' comparative achievement as well as individual attainment.

3. Relies on both teacher and student input.

4. Focuses on the process and the products of learning.

5. Is based on multiple forms of assessment.

6. Includes students' self-assessments, the teacher's, and the collaborative effort stemming from their interaction.

7. Features the students' best work; shows what the students know and how they progress over time.

8. Explores a broad range of activities and is multidimensional in scope.

9. Portrays a complete picture of individual students.

B. Dynamic Assessment

Dynamic assessment involves coaching to assist children's performance and learning in a test-teach-retest paradigm. The examiner actively interacts with each child.

1. The procedure allows children to exhibit their skills over extended periods of time.

2. Goal of dynamic assessment is to rule out lack of experience as a reason for a deficiency.

3. The child, with the mediator, learns how to think, learn, solve problems, apply learning to other situations, and to self-regulate behavior.

4. Typical students improve dramatically on a retest after coaching, with children with language disability not improving greatly.

5. The behaviors the mediator is assessing include:

   a. **Attention:** whether the child independently maintains attention throughout length of task.

   b. **Self-awareness/regulation:** whether the child is aware of correctness of response/performance and shows systematic approach to new tasks.

   c. **Motivation:** whether the child shows persistence for the task (Pena, Quinn, & Iglesias, 1992).

6. On applied modifications to *Clinical Evaluation of Language Fundamentals-Revised* (CELF-R) to typical bilingual students with fluent English proficiency. The students scored significantly higher on the modified test (Franklin & Saenz, 1994).

7. In dynamic assessment at the word level, significant differences were found in the performance between children with mild language impairments and normal children (Pena, Quinn, & Iglesias, 1992).

8. Roseberry and Connell (1991) found the performance of children with typical and atypical language to be different on a novel or unknown targeted learning task. Therefore, the assumption is that language impairments could be identified using this type of testing task, but Restrepo (1995) used a novel based learning task and found no difference in the performance of children with typical and atypical language.

XII. INTERPRETERS

An interpreter is defined by Langdon and Cheng (1992) as conveying information from one language to the other in the spoken language and the translator employs writing. Appendix G is a listing of English-Spanish terminology that may be used to orient the interpreter.

A. Recommended Linguistic and Educational Qualifications (Kayser, 1993)

   1. High school diploma or its equivalent;

2. Adequate communication skills;

3. Ability to relate to the clinical population being served;

4. High degree of oral proficiency and literacy in both English and the minority language;

5. Ability to shift styles depending on the dialect used;

6. Ability to memorize and retain chunks of information while interpreting;

7. Command of the medical, educational, speech-language pathology, and audiology terminology.

B. **The standards for language proficiency** may have to be flexible, so that interpreter-assistants who are not completely literate in their home language can still be used for a limited number of useful activities.

C. **The American Speech-Language-Hearing Association** (ASHA) (1985) recommends that interpreters can be recruited through referral from professional foreign language schools and university language programs.

   1. Sources for recruiting interpreters also include local churches, other settings, foreign missions, and international cultural centers.

   2. Volunteer interpreters or translators may require training and additional preparation time for a particular conference or assessment session.

D. **The interpreter's activities** should be reviewed and assigned by the clinician for three areas: assessment, conference, and intervention phases.

   1. **Assessment**

      a. The interpreter must have:
         (1) Understanding of the rationale, procedures, and information that is obtained from tests.
         (2) Opportunity and time to review the test questions and examine them for cultural relevancy.

    b. Duties under the supervision of the clinician may include:
      (1) Administering a variety of tests
      (2) Obtaining questionnaire information
      (3) Eliciting language samples
      (4) Participating in speech-language and hearing screenings
      (5) Scheduling activities
      (6) Preparing charts
      (7) Recording and displaying test data

    c. Training for the interpreter in the administration of tests is necessary, as well as conducting reliability checks to ensure that the interpreter has the skill necessary to administer and score each test accurately and reliably.

2. Conferences

There are four common types of changes (errors) in information that an interpreter may make during a conference session that a clinician should be alert to.

    a. The interpreter may omit the clinician's messages. The omission of information may be at the word, phrase, or sentence level. The reasons for omitting the utterance may be that the interpreter does not believe a specific word is important to relay, or he or she may not understand the English word, phrase, or sentence. The interpreter may just forget to include the utterance.

    b. The interpreter may add extra words, phrases, or sentences not said by the clinician to editorialize.

    c. Additions also may occur because extra words are needed to explain a concept that is difficult to translate. The interpreter may not remember the specific message or be confused with words that sound alike; therefore, other words, phrases, or sentences are substituted.

    d. Transformations by interpreters are changes in the word order of what was actually said (Langdon, 1992). A interpreter-assistant may be concerned about a client's comprehension and, therefore, elaborate, simplify, and reword.

    e. To assist the interpreter during conferences, the professional should:

(1) Keep language simple and short, without professional jargon and extra wording,

(2) Watch the interpreter's body language, and

(3) Listen for the use of too many or too few words compared to the clinician's utterances.

f. The interpreter can also help the process and, therefore, should:

(1) Be free to request that the speaker rephrase unclear messages,

(2) Listen carefully: take notes, consult a dictionary, and

(3) Know one's own limitations as an interpreter

3. **Intervention**

The interpreter-assistant should not write, develop, or modify the client's intervention plan in any way without the recommendation, guidance, and approval of the supervising clinician.

a. Training should include review of the intervention materials with the interpreter, discussion of the purpose of the procedures, and demonstration by the clinician.

b. Actual supervision of intervention sessions will depend on the client's type of impairment and severity in addition to the experience and competency level of the interpreter-assistant. This may range from 100% supervision at the initiation of intervention to 10% once the assistant and clinician are comfortable with the caseload and procedures.

E. **Suggestions on interactions** of clinician and interpreter for each conference, assessment, and intervention session by Langdon (1992) include:

1. **Briefing** is the clinician's opportunity to meet with the interpreter and to review the general purpose of the session, whether it is for an initial conference or testing session, which also allows the interpreter time to review materials and ask questions.

2. **Interaction**

3. **Debriefing** follows the interaction and allows the clinician and interpreter to discuss the client's responses and errors, plus the interpreter's observations, test scoring, and any difficulties during the session.

XIII. CONCLUSION

There are a number of tests, observation procedures, taxonomies for pragmatics, questionnaires, and ethnographic interviews that can be part of the assessment of children who are bilingual. We know that children who speak typically when they enter kindergarten probably lose their ability to speak the home language as they learn English. These children are at high risk for referral for speech and language assessment. The important part of any evaluation is the prereferral, the child's history, and parental concerns. The teacher may have concerns about academics. The history of education in the United States indicates that 50% of Hispanics will fail and drop out of school. Speech-language pathologists must be aware that language concerns within the classroom should be viewed critically, with special understanding that one in two Hispanic children do not understand what is happening in these classrooms because of second language acquisition and cultural influences on classroom interactions that may be unfamiliar to the child.

CHAPTER

5

Language Analysis

Because tests are not developed specifically for Spanish speaking populations, published tests may have to be adapted to conform to the Spanish dialect of a region, and clinicians may need to modify their procedures to elicit the best possible performance from a Hispanic child. The clinician needs speech and language samples to determine if a child, indeed, exhibits a speech and language impairment. This chapter provides information on elicitation procedures, developmental data for Spanish-speaking children, and analysis procedures for use in language sample analysis.

I. ELICITATION OF LANGUAGE SAMPLES

Kayser and Restrepo, 1995 offer some considerations:

A. **The Hispanic child may be reared** to believe that he or she is not an equal conversational partner to an adult (Heath, 1986). Therefore, an Hispanic child may not easily converse with a speech-language pathologist.

B. A minimum of three language samples is recommended— clinician–child, peer–child, and parent–child— if possible.

C. There should be a variety of elicitation procedures used to obtain the language sample.

D. There are a number of recommended elicitation procedures (see Table 5–1) for techniques and age levels.

E. A free play or a conversational format is less demanding on a child's language than a story retelling task, suggest Restrepo, Chasteen, and Bejarano (Unpublished manuscript).

F. A structured language elicitation task yielded higher performance in Spanish-speaking children with normal language than a standardized language test suggests (R. T. Anderson, 1996).

G. When a structured language task is used, the clinician must know how typical children will respond to the task, before administering it to children with language impairment (R. T. Anderson, 1996).

II. IMPORTANT FEATURES OF SPANISH PHONOLOGY

A. Spanish phonology is made up of 19 consonants and 2 semi-vowels, as compared to 24 consonants and 2 semivowels in English.

B. Many of the Spanish consonants are unaspirated and there is a perceptually different production of the consonants, as compared to English.

C. Spanish contains 10 syllabic nuclei (vowels) compared to 17 frequently occurring nuclei in English (Stockwell , 1965).

D. Rules governing the combinations of sounds within each of the languages differ. Spanish has a simpler phonological rule system than English.

Table 5-1. Elicitation Techniques

Technique	Description	Application	Examples	Age Level
Probe	Student responds to open- or closed-ended questions	Elicits yes/no or short response	Why did he do that? Does he cook at home?	Children/Adults
Description	Describes an object	Use a variety of stimuli; toys for children pictures for adults	Tell me about the toy/picture	Children/Adults
Narration	Describes a sequence of events	Can talk about play event, retell cartoons just seen, wordless picture books, comic books, or folktale.	What's she doing?	Children/Adults
Interpretation	Provides meanings of stimuli	Person interprets motives of characters, artist's intended meaning, music's message.	Why would the monster want to?	Adolescents/Adults
Expression	Reacts personally to a stimulus	Present several toys and ask why the toy was chosen, ask for story with conflict, relate it to a meaningful real incident.	Tell me about the time you were embarrassed in class.	Children/Adults
Explication	Provides information about a process or procedure	Verbal directions to get to a neighborhood, show street map and ask how to get from one point to next. Also building a house or toy, cooking foods.	Tell me step-by-step.	Children/Adults

(continued)

Table 5-1. Elicitation Techniques *(continued)*

Technique	Description	Application	Examples	Age Level
Elaboration	Must expand on topic	Ask for elaboration on topic already introduced in interaction.	Tell me more.	Children/Adults
Role-playing	Must use language appropriate for situation.	Suggest an imaginary situation parent/teacher caught you fighting, arguing with sibling, asking for a date, clearing up a misunderstanding, apologizing to friend, forgetting a meeting.	Excuse me. May I help you?	Children/Adults
Games/problem solving	Must verbalize answer to problems.	Counting games, identifying errors or inconsistencies, guessing games, telling how a toy/machine works.	What's wrong with it?	Children/Adults
Sustained production	Produces a stream of uninterrupted language or topics.	Recites as many words as possible without stopping.	I want you to say as many words in English as you can.	Children/Adults
Paraphrase	Asked to express an idea another way.	Express an idea differently without changing the meaning.	Say this differently.	Adolescents/Adults

Source: From "Language Samples: Elicitation and Analysis," by H. Kayser and M. A. Restrepo. In *Bilingual Speech-Language Pathology: An Hispanic Focus* (pp. 272–273), by H. Kayser (Ed.), 1995, San Diego: Singular Publishing Group, Inc. Copyright 1995 by Singular Publishing Group Inc. Reprinted with permission.

Table 5–2. Spanish Phoneme Development

	Acevedo (1989) (Mexican-American)	Jimenez (1987) (Mexican-American)	Linares (1981) (Mexican)	Terrero (1979) (Venezuelan)
m	3;6	3;7	3	3;1
n	3;6	3;7	3	4;1
p	3;6	3;3	3	3;1
b	3;6	3;3	6	3;9
B	—	—	6	—
k	3;6	3;7	3	3;1
g	3;6	4;7	3	5;5
t	4;0	3;3	3	3;1
d	4;0	4;7	4	4;9
d	>5;6	—	4	>5;5
f	3;6	4;3	4	4;9
j	4;6	3;11	3	5;1
l	4;6	3;11	3	4;5 (M)*
				>5;5 (F)*
x	5;0	4;7	3	4;1 (M)
				>5;5 (F)
t	5;0	4;7	4	5;1
s	<5;6	5;7	6	>5;5
r	3;6	4;7	4	>5;1 (M)
				5;5 (F)
rr	>5;6	>5;7	6	>5;5
ñ	3;6	4;11	3	4;9
w	3;6	3;7	5	—
ng	—	—	3	—

The ages (in years; months) indicate the point at which the subjects had mastered the respective phonemes, with mastery being at the 90% level. < means "younger than." > refers to "older than."

*M and F refer to medial and final positions, respectively. These differences were reported if they spanned more than two age groups. Those ages not designated as corresponding to word position indicate the age at which the phonemes are mastered in all positions in which they occur.

Source: From D. M. Paulson, *Phonological Systems of Spanish-Speaking Texas Preschoolers* (master's thesis), by D. P. Mann, 1991, Texas Christian University, Fort Worth, TX. Copyright 1991 by D. P. Mann. Reprinted with permission.

E. **Spanish phoneme development** from Paulson (1991) is in Table 5–2.

F. **Spanish-speaking children** may occasionally exhibit cluster reduction, unstressed syllable deletion, stridency deletion, and tap/trill/r/ deviations as noted by Goldstein (1995) (see Table 5–3 and Table 5–4).

Table 5-3. Percentage of Spanish-Speaking Children Exhibiting Phonological Processes

Process*	Meza (1983)	Goldstein (1993)
Cluster reduction	100	83
Unstressed syllable deletion	100	81
Stopping	80	93
Palatal fronting	40	20
Liquid simplification	95	94
Assimilation	95	87

*Only processes targeted in both studies are listed.
Source: From "Spanish Phonological Development," by B. A. Goldstein. In *Bilingual Speech-Language Pathology: An Hispanic Focus* (p. 26), by H. Kayser (Ed.), (1995), San Diego: Singular Publishing Group, Inc. Copyright 1995 by Singular Publishing Group Inc. Reprinted with permission.

III. FEATURES OF SPANISH MORPHOSYNTACTIC DEVELOPMENT

A. **Spanish-speaking children use single words** before age 2, two-word utterances by age 2, and simple three-word constructions by age 3.

B. **Spanish-speaking children ask questions** and use compound sentences with conjunctions by age 4½.

C. **By age 4½ a Spanish-speaking** child is likely using approximately 38 different syntactic structures (E. Garcia & Gonzalez, 1984).

D. **Spanish-speaking children** have difficulty with gender and number agreement as late as age 6 (E. Garcia & Gonzalez, 1984; E. Garcia, Maez, & Gonzalez, 1984).

E. **The acquisition of article and gender agreement** may be affected by the complexity in use, the influence of English, and the possibility of language attrition.

F. **Dialect variations that are used by the parent** may be mirrored by children. (R. T. Anderson, 1995).

Table 5–4. Considerations for Phonological Assessment and Treatment of Spanish-Speaking Children

---

I. **Considerations for Phonological Assessment** (after Bernthal & Bankson, 1993, pp. 222–223).
   A. Use an assessment tool designed specifically to assess Spanish-speaking children
   B. Take the child's dialect into account
   C. Describe the phonological status of an individual
   D. Determine if the child's phonological system is sufficiently different from normal development to warrant intervention
   E. Determine treatment direction
   F. Make predictive and prognostic statements relative to phonological change with or without intervention
   G. Monitor change in phonological performance
   H. Identify factors that may be related to the presence or maintenance of a phonological disability
II. **Phonological Assessment Tools for Spanish-Speaking Children**
   A. *Austin Spanish Articulation Test* (Carrow, 1974)
   B. *Assessment of Phonological Processes—Spanish* (Hodson, 1986)
   C. *Assessment of Phonological Disabilities* (Iglesias, 1978)
   D. *Southwest Spanish Articulation Test* (Toronto, 1977)
III. **General Considerations in the Treatment of Phonological Disorders** (after Stoel-Gammon & Dunn, 1985, pp. 166–167)
   A. Developing a treatment plan based on underlying factors that contribute to etiology of the disorder (e.g., auditory status, structural adequacy, and motoric abilities)
   B. Consider each child as an individual
   C. Use normal acquisition data as a guide to planning treatment goals
   D. Have a philosophical framework (e.g., phone mastery vs. phonological processes)
   E. Teach the child to monitor responses
   F. Measure progress with an initial baseline, intermittent testing to determine progress, and testing for generalization.
   G. Consider when selecting targets:
      1. The phones in the child's repertoire
      2. The frequency of occurrence of the phone in the language
      3. Age of acquisition and ease of production of the phone
      4. Stimulability
      5. Age of client

Source: From "Spanish Phonological Development," by B. A. Goldstein. In *Bilingual Speech-Language Pathology: An Hispanic Focus* (p. 30), by H. Kayser (Ed.), 1995, San Diego: Singular Publishing Group, Inc. Copyright 1995 by Singular Publishing Group Inc. Reprinted with permission.

Table 5–5. Spanish Personal Pronoun Development

	Age Range (years; month)			
	2;0	*2;6*	*3;0*	*2;6*
Yo	———————			
Tu	———————			
El/ella	————————————			
Me	————————————			
Te	——————————————————			
La/lo	——————————————————			
Se	——————————————————			

Note: Clitic pronouns include both reflexive and nonreflexive uses. Plural forms were evidenced in Schum et al., (1992) at approximately 2;6 years for subject pronoun forms.
Source: From "Spanish Morphological and Syntactic Development," by R. T. Anderson. In *Bilingual Speech-Language Pathology: An Hispanic Focus* (p. 61), by H. Kayser (Ed.), 1995, San Diego: Singular Publishing Group, Inc. Copyright 1995 by Singular Publishing Group Inc. Reprinted with permission.

G. **Compare L2 morphosyntactic errors** as they apply to normal developmental morphosyntactic patterns found in L1 as well as possible L2 transference (R. T. Anderson, 1997).

H. **Spanish-speaking children** with language impairments:

1. Had most commonly had errors of omission of prepositions and articles, person agreement for verbs, and gender agreement for articles, as found by Restrepo (1995).

2. Produced errors in 24% of their articles, compared to 2% in the normal group (Restrepo, Chasteen, Bustelo, & Matute, 1996).

3. Only 2% produced errors, in use of verbs (Restrepo, Chasteen, Bustelo, & Matute, 1996).

I. **Developmental data** concerning typical Spanish-speaking children and the use of morphosyntactic forms is necessary. (R. T. Anderson, 1995; Hornak, Trujillo, & Kayser, 1996) (see Tables 5–5, 5–6, 5–7, 5–8, and 5–9).

Table 5–6. Age Ranges for the Development of Verb Inflection in Spanish-Speaking Children

	Age Range (years; months)								
Tense	2;0	2;6	3;0	3;6	4;0	4;6	5;0	5;6	6;0
Present indicative	———								
Simple preterit	———								
Imperative	———								
Copulas	———								
Present progressive	———								
Compound preterit			———————————————						
Periphrastic future				——————————————					
Imperfect preterit				—————————					
Present subjunctive				————————————————————————					
Past progressive					———————				
Past subjunctive						——————————————————			

Note: Beginnings of line indicate initial age of appearance when the specific tense was noted. The lines demarcate ranges in the acquisition of the forms.

Source: From "Spanish Morphological and Syntactic Development," by R. T. Anderson. In *Bilingual Speech-Language Pathology: An Hispanic Focus* (p. 58), by H. Kayser (Ed.), 1995, San Diego: Singular Publishing Group, Inc. Copyright 1995 by Singular Publishing Group Inc. Reprinted with permission.

IV. ANALYSIS PROCEDURES FOR LANGUAGE SAMPLES

There are several initial procedures that may document a Spanish-speaking child's expressive language competencies for syntax. Only one of the procedures described here has normative data collected from Puerto Rican children (Toronto, 1976). Each of these procedures may be used as descriptive measures and then compared to the developmental data reported in Tables 5–5 through 5–9.

A. Mean Length Response (MLR)

R. T. Anderson (1995) and Kayser and Restrepo (1995) suggest the use of MLR instead of mean length of utterance (MLU) for Spanish speaking

Table 5–7. Summary of Developmental Data for Morphosyntactic Development in Spanish-Speaking Children

Age Range	Verb Morphology	Noun Phrase Elaboration	Prepositional Phrases	Syntactic Structure

2;0–3;0	Present indicative
	Simple preterit
	Imperative
	Periphrastic**
	  future
	Copulas *ser/estar*
		Indefinite and
		  definite articles
		Article gender
		Plural /s/
		Plural /es/
			en
			con
			para
			a
			de
				Sentences with
				  copula verbs
				Use of clitic
				  direct object
				Reflexive
				  constructions
				(S)VO
				  sentences
				Yes/no
				  questions
				Negative with
				  no before
				  verb phrase
				Imperative
				  sentences
				Wh-questions
				  qué
				  quién
				  dónde
				  para qué
				  cuándo
				  por qué
				  cómo
				  de quién
				  con quién
				Embedded
				  sentences
				Embedded
				  direct object

3;0-4;0	Imperfect preterit
	Past progressive
	Ir progressive
	Past/present
	Compound preterit
	Present subjunctive
		Grammatical
		  gender in nouns
		  and adjectives
		Use of quantifiers
			hasta
			entre
			desde
			sobre
				Wh-questions
				  established
				Use of full set
				  of negatives
				Subjunctive
				  clauses
				Embedding

4;0-5;0	Past subjunctive
	Present perfect
	  indicative
		Gender in clitic
		3rd person
		  pronouns		

*Preterite expresses an action that was completed at some time in the past.

**Periphrastic is the use of a longer form.

Source: From "Spanish Morphological and Syntactic Development," by R. T. Anderson. In *Bilingual Speech-Language Pathology: An Hispanic Focus* (p. 57), by H. Kayser (Ed.), 1995, San Diego: Singular Publishing Group, Inc. Copyright 1995 by Singular Publishing Group Inc. Reprinted with permission.

children. MLR should be used for younger children. The child's responsiveness to the clinician and the clinician's skills in eliciting the language sample will affect the representativeness of the child's language abilities. Therefore, the language sample should be examined before an MLR is calculated.

1. Check on the representativeness of the MLR by looking at:

    a. **High rate of imitation.** May need to analyze the imitative and spontaneous utterances separately.

    b. **Frequent self-repetitions within a speech turn.** May need to analyze with and without repetitions to determine if this produces a difference in the MLR.

    c. **High proportion of question-answers** in the child's speech. This may produce shorter responses in child's utterances. It may be necessary to obtain another language sample.

    d. **Frequent routines** such as counting, alphabet, and so on. The MLR may be biased with the inclusion of these routines. Compute with and without the routines and determine if it makes a difference.

2. Divide the language sample into utterances. An utterance is marked by a rising or falling intonation contour and a terminal pause (J. Miller, 1981).

3. The number of words per utterance are counted and averaged across the total number of utterances.

B. Terminal units (TU) should be used for older children to determine the complexity of utterances.

1. Defined as a main clause and all its dependent clauses.

    a. Each clause has its own main verb.

    b. Clauses may be conjoined to the main clause by coordinating or subordinating conjunction.
       (1) Coordinating conjunctions include: *y, y luego, entonces, pero, o, ni, tambien,* and *sin embargo.*

Table 5–8. Morphological and Syntactical Structures for Children From Monolingual and Bilingual Environments

Syntactical and Morphological Markers	Monolingual Environment (Gudeman, 1981; Kernan & Blount, 1966; Merino, 1976; Olarte, 1985; Romero, 1985)	Bilingual Environment (Brisk, 1972, 1976; Cohen, 1980; Dale 1980; Garcia, 1988; *Gonzalez, 1978, 1980; Maez, 1983; Parra, 1982)
Present indicative (El muchacho hace—The boy does)	Merino—4.0 Olarte—2.9	Cohen—4.0 Garcia—2.0–4.5 *Gonzalez—2.0–2.6 Maez—1.6–2.0
1st person singular (Yo hago.—I do.)		*Gonzalez—2.6
2nd person singular (Tú haces.—You do.)		*Gonzalez—2.6
3rd person singular (Él hizo.—He did.)		*Gonzalez—2.6
3rd person plural (Ellos hacen.—They do.)		*Gonzalez—2.6
Present progressive (El muchacho hace.—The boy does.)	Olarte—3.1	Cohen—3.0 Garcia—2.6–4.5 *Gonzalez—2.0–2.6
Progressive participle/gerund (Yo estoy haciendo.—I am doing.)	Romero—3.6–4.7	
Progressive past (Estaba haciendo.—Was doing.)		*Gonzalez—2.6–4.0
Present perfect/auxiliary present (Ella ha hecho.—She has done.)	Merino—4.0 Kernan & Blount—11.0–12.0	Garcia—4.5 *Gonzalez—3.0–4.6

Grammatical form		
Preterit regular*** (Yo hice.—I did.)	Merino—4.0 Gudeman—7.1–9.0 Kernan & Blount—11.0–12.0 **Olarte—2.6 Romero—3.6–4.7	Cohen—3.0–4.0 Dale—5.0 Garcia—4.5 *Gonzalez—2.0–2.6 Maez—1.10 (3rd person)
Preterit irregular (Yo supe.—I knew.)	Merino—4.0–5.0 Kernan & Blount—11.0–12.0	
Imperfect indicative (hacìa—did)	Romero—3.6–4.7	Cohen—4.0 Garcia—3.0–4.5 *Gonzalez—2.9– 3.3
Future or periphrastic future (harè/va a hacer—I will do)	Olarte—3.8 Romero—3.6–4.7	Brisk—5.0 Cohen—4.0 Garcia—2.6 *Gonzalez—2.6
Conditional (Si el niño no lo hace, nadie lo hace.—If the boy doesn't do it, no one will.)	Merino—6.0	Brisk—5.0 Cohen—3.5 Garcia—3.0 (Emerging) *Gonzalez—3.0–4.0
Present subjunctive (Quiero que Maria lo haga.—I want Maria to do it.)	Merino—4.0	Cohen—3.0–7.0 Garcia—3.0–4.5 *Gonzalez—2.6–4.0
Past subjunctive (Yo haya hecho.—I would have done.)		Garcia—4.5 *Gonzalez—3.3–4.6
Copula (ser/estar—is)		Garcia—3.0 *Gonzalez—2.0 (3rd Person)
Imperative consisting of verb form. (haga—do)	Romero—3.6–4.7	*Gonzalez—2.0 Maez—1.6

(continued)

Table 5–8. Morphological and Syntactical Structures for Children From Monolingual and Bilingual Environments *(continued)*

Syntactical and Morphological Markers	Monolingual Environment (Gudeman, 1981; Kernan & Blount, 1966; Merino, 1976; Olarte, 1985; Romero, 1985)	Bilingual Environment (Brisk, 1972, 1976; Cohen, 1980; Dale 1980; Garcia, 1988; *Gonzalez, 1978, 1980; Maez, 1983; Parra, 1982)
Imperatives verb + indirect object (No lo hagas.—Do not do it.) verb + reflexive pronoun (Hazlo hija.—Do it daughter.)		Garcia—4.5 *Gonzalez—2.6
Imperatives: verb + indirect/direct object (Hazlo.—do it.) or verb + reflexive + direct object pronoun (Hazlo tù.—Do it yourself.)		Garcia—4.5 *Gonzalez—2.9
Passives (El vestido fue hecho por la mamà.— The dress was made by the mother.)	Merino—7.0–8.0 Gudeman—12.4–Adult	
Prepositions (en, sobre, debajo, detras—in, on, under, behind.)		Garcia—3.0
Short plurals /s/	Merino—4.0 Kernan & Blount—5.0– 7.0 Gudeman—7.1–9.0 Olarte—2.11	Dale—5.0
Long plurals /es/	Merino—4.0 Kernan & Blount—11.0–12.0 Olarte—3.2	Dale—8.0
Possessive, constructive (de su padre, del papà, etc.—his father's)	Olarte—2.11	*Gonzalez—2.6–3.0

Interrogatives (dónde, qué, cómo, quién, cuál, por qué, para qué—where, what, how, who, which, why, for what)		*Gonzalez—2.0 (Donde, Que, Por Que) *Gonzalez—2.6–4.0 (Quien, Cuando, Como, and Para que)
Qualifying primitive adjective (bonito—pretty)		Garcia—3.0–6.0 Parra—2.0–2.11
Possessive adjective (En el vestido de la princesa.—On the princess' dress.)		Parra—3.0–3.11
Gender, noun adjectives—substantivization (los caballos, las muchachas la camisa blanca—the horses, the girls, the white shirt)	Merino—4.0 Olarte—3.2	*Gonzalez—2.9–4.0 Parra—2.0–12.0
Yes/No questions in full sentence form (No lo hizò hoy.—Used as response. —He/She didn't do it today.)		*Gonzalez—2.6–4.0
Locative adverbs (recio—fast)		Garcia—3.0 (Emerging) Gonzalez—2.9
Conjunctive (El niño lo hizò y la muchacha no lo hizò.—The boy did it and the girl did not do it.)		Garcia—4.5 *Gonzalez—2.6–4.0
Negatives (<u>No</u> lo haga.—Don't do it.)		Garcia—3.0 *Gonzalez—2.0–2.6
Pronouns (èl, ella, ellos—he, she, they)		Garcia—3.0
Reflexive pronoun (Me lo hizò.—He/She did it for me.)		*Gonzalez—2.0

*Gonzalez: First age indicates age of emergence and second age indicates established age of acquisition. All other investigators only reported established age of acquisition.

**Olarte stated only emerging age.

***Preterit expresses an action that was completed at some time in the past.

Table 5–9. Investigated Studies

Name of Researcher	Location of Study	Ages Studied	Method of Data Elicitation
Brisk (1972)	United States—Urban/rural New Mexico	5.0—5.11	Guided conversation
Cohen (1980)	United States—San Francisco	2.11—7.1	Guided conversation
Dale (1980)	United States—Miami	5.0—8.0	Berko Nonsense Words
Garcia (1988)	United States—Urban/rural areas	3.0—4.11	Criterion referenced instrument elicited spontaneous procedure using stimuli photographs (SPELT-P)
Gonzalez (1978)	United States—Texas	2.0—5.0	Guided conversation
Gudeman (1981)	Panama—Rural	4.0—Adult	Berko Nonsense Words
Kernan & Blount (1966)	Mexico—Rural Ciudad Guzman, Jalisco	5.0—12.0	Berko Nonsense Words
Maez (1983)	Location not stated	1.6—2.0	Language samples and mean length of utterance (MLU)
Merino (1976, 1992)	Mexico—Oaxaca	4.0—8.0	Comprehension and production with pictures
Olarte (1985)	Columbia	2.6—4.2	Cued responses to comprehension and expression
Parra (1982)	United States	2.0—12.0	Structured conversation with pictures
Romero (1985)	Puerto Rico	3.6—4.7	Story retelling and structured conversation

(2) Subordinating conjunctions include: *eso cuál, quien, qué, dónde, despues, aunqué, cómo, cómo si, antes, si, desde qué, hasta qué, cuándo, mientras, and a menos qué.*

2. **TU calculation**

   a. Two clauses joined by a subordinating conjunction equals one TU.

   b. Two clauses joined by a coordinating conjunction with the subject of second clause deleted equals one TU.

   c. Two clauses joined by a coordinating conjunction with the subject stated in the second clause equals two TU.

V. DEVELOPMENTAL SENTENCE TYPES (DST)

An analysis procedure for the younger child was developed by Lee (1974). It does not give an overall score but does allow the clinician to arrive at a judgment regarding the child's language development.

A. Requires a 100-utterance language sample with more than 50% of the utterances incomplete (lacking a subject and verb).

1. Clinician charts the number of single words, two-word combinations, multiword constructions, and complete sentences in the language sample.

2. Percentage of occurrence for each category is computed (e.g., percentage of single words, two-word combinations, etc.).

B. This type of analysis provides documentation of language growth.

C. Table 5–10 provides Spanish-speaking examples and Table 5–11 a DST analysis form (Kayser, 1997).

VI. THE DEVELOPMENTAL ASSESSMENT OF SPANISH GRAMMAR (DASG)

The DASG (Toronto, 1976) is an adaptation of developmental sentence scoring (Lee, 1974). It is limited in its range of analyses, but it does provide an

Table 5–10. DST—Developmental Sentence Types

	Noun	Designator	Descriptive Items	Verb	Vocabulary Item
One Word	carro papa gatito camion mama muñeca galleta niña tortilla Basic sentence elaborations: Plural: libros, niños, hombres Basic sentence modifications: Pronoun: yo, algo, nadie Question: Libro? Carro? Camión?	Aquí, acá, allí, allá este, esta, ese, esa, aquí, aquélla lo, la Basic sentence elaborations: Plural: esos, esas, aquéllos, aquéllas Basic sentence modifications: Question: Eso? Aquélla? Aquí? Allá?	Grande, bonita, roto, azul uno, dos, un en, sobre, fuera de, arriba Basic sentence elaborations: Plural: grandes, bonitas Basic sentence modifications: Pronoun: mi, mis, su, sus Question: Grande? bonita?	duermo, comes, anda, caen, gritamos (mira, espera, escucha = imperative sentence) Basic sentence elaborations: Verb elaboration: se cayó, parate Basic sentence modifications: Negative: no come, no lloro Question: Mira? Juegas ?	si, no, bien, shh, oye, hola, adios, ay! Basic sentence elaborations: Adverb: otra vez, ahora, tambien Basic sentence modifications: Question: Qué? Verdad? Quién? Como? Porque? Dónde? Conjunction: y, e

	Noun Elaboration	Designative Elaboration	Predicative	Verbal Elaboration	Fragments
Two Words	Noun phrase Article: un carro, el camion Possessive: Jose mochila, Alma sueter Quantifier: un carro, dos niños Adjective: carro grande, camión sucio Attributive: osito, carro policia Basic sentence elaborations: Plural: los carros, los camións Additive: carro camión, mama papa Adverb: ahora carro, camión tambien Subject-object: papa pelota, perro plato Subject-locative: carro garaje, mama silla Basic sentence modifications: Pronoun: mi camion, su galleta Negative: carro no, camión no, eso no Question: Cual carro? Otro camión? Conjunction: (carro y caso...)	Designator + noun carro aqui, camión alla, ese dulce, aquel camión, aquélla muñeca Basic sentence elaboration: Plural: estos carros, allá camiónes Adverb: (eso otra vez = noun + adverb) (aquélla ahora, aquí otra vez = fragments) Basic sentence modifications: Pronoun: aquí algo, alla uno Negative: (eso no = noun + negative) (aquí no, alla no = fragments) Question: Aquél carro? Cual este? Conjunctions: (y este = noun + conj.) (y aquí, y alla = fragments)	Noun + descriptive item carro roto, camión sucio, helado alla, muñeca aquí Basic sentence elaborations: Plural: carros aqui, muñecas bonitas Basic sentence modifications: Pronoun: aquella bonita, algo aqui, otro sobre Question: Carro roto? Lo acabo? Carro donde? Quien alla? Que aqui?	Verb + object: choca carro Verb + locative: sientate silla (Noun + verb = sentence, bebe duerme se cayo, ese va) Basic sentence elaborations: Verb elaboration: choco carro Plural: come galletas, veo carros Adverb: comen ahora, cae tambien Basic sentence modifications: Pronoun: lo ves, buscalo Negative: no cae, no va Question: Lo ves? Te vas? Donde va? Que halla? (Quien va? Que viene = sentence) Conjunction: y durmiendo Infinitive: irme, acostarse	Basic sentence elaborations: Prepositional phrase: para papa, en carro Plural: abajo sillas, en carros Adverb: demiado grande, aqui otra vez Basic sentence modifications: Pronoun: a ti, entrelo Negative: pega no, aqui no Question: Er ese? Conjunction: y grande, pero sucio, y aquí	

Constructions				
Noun phrase *mi carro grande, una caja azul,* Noun phrase + prepositional phrase *el carro enfrente, el gato en la silla* Quantifier + prepositional phrase *todos de esos, algunos de los otros carros* Basic sentence elaborations: Plural: *algunos otros carros* Adverb: *ahora el carro, el otro camión tambien* Additive: *el carro el camión* Subject-object: *el perro otro hueso* Subject-locative: *el carro el garaje* Basic sentence modifications: Pronoun: *su otro camión, todo mio* Negative: *el carro no, eso no* Question: *El otro carro? El niño tambien?* *Cual carro grande?* *Cuantas galletas?* *Cual otro? Quien?* Conjunction: *y el carro, carro y camión*	Designator + noun phrase *aquí otro carro, allá un camión* *eso un carro rojo, aquel camión mío* Basic Sentence elaborations: Plural: *aquí algunos carros, esos carros grandes* Adverb: *allá el carro tambien, aquí carro ahora* Additive: *allá Mama Papa* Basic sentence modifications: Pronoun: *aquel carro de alguien, aquí su carro* Negative: *aquel carro no eso no un camión* Question: *Aquel un carro? Eso un camion? Quién aquel nino? Que aquello?* Conjunction: *aquí un carro y camión*	Noun phrase + descriptive item *el carro roto, un camión sucio, otro carro allá, un camión aquí, carro en garaje* Basic sentence elaborations: Plural: *todos carros rotos* Adverb: *carro aquí tambien, camión sucio ahora* Double locator: *carro allá afuera* Basic sentence modification: Pronoun: *el niño travieso* Negative: *eso no roto* Question: *Quién en carro? Qué color el carro? Qué aquí adentro?* Conjunction: *carro y camión aquí*	Verb + object: *come la galleta* Verb + locative: *pon la mesa* (Noun phrase + verb = sentence: *el carro va, un niño come*) Basic sentence elaborations: Verb elaboration: *correen granero* Adverb: *mira carro ahora, cabe tambien* Basic sentence modification: Pronoun: *lo quiro ahora* Negative: *no cae* Question: *Mira aquéllo? Come las galletas? Donde ponga el carro? Qué saque? Qué halle aquí? Qué hace al carro?* Conjunction: *y halla carro* Infinitive: *quiere verlo, irse a casa, necesito hallarlo.*	Words in series: *uno, dos, tres, perro, vaca, gat* Basic sentence elaborations: Prepositional phrase: *en el carro, para el niño* Plural: *sobre las sillas* Adverb: *en carro tambien, allá atras* Basic sentence modifications: Pronoun: *en mi cabeza* Negative: *en eso no* Question: *En eso tambien?* *En el carro?* Conjunction: *y para mi*

Source: Adapted from *Developmental Sentence Analysis* (pp. 86–87) by L. L. Lee, 1974, Evanston, IL: Northwestern University Press. Copyright 1974 by Northwestern University Press. Adapted with permission.

Table 5–11. Developmental Sentence Types Form

Name: _____ Date: _____

Birth Date: _____ C.A.: _____

Examiner: _____

Single Words: _____
2-Word combinations: _____
Constructions: _____
Sentences: _____

	Noun	Designator	Descriptive Item	Verb	Vocabulary Item
One Word					
	Noun Elaboration	*Designative Elaboration*	*Predicative Elaboration*	*Verbal Elaboration*	*Fragments*
Two Words					
Construction					

indication of syntactic development in children. Kayser and Restrepo (1995) suggest that clinicians should obtain new norms and obtain discriminant validity or use it for descriptive purposes.

A. Scoring

1. The DASG requires a language sample taken from an adult-child interaction. A total of 50 consecutive utterances are used for scoring from a corpus of 100 utterances.

2. Only count complete sentences containing subject or implied optional pronoun (subject plus a verb) (e.g., "El viene," or "Viene").

3. Count independent clauses when they are part of fragmented sentences, (e.g., "Aquí, pero no se lo que es").

4. Do not count dependent clauses or indirect questions used to answer questions (e.g., A: "qué le dice la mama?" C: "Qué venga a comer." Not counted. A: "Qué quiere saber el nino?" C: "Donde va?" Not counted).

5. Do not count incomplete or unintelligible sentences (Figure 5–1).

6. If a sentence is repeated, count one time only in the sample.

7. If stereotypical phrases/words are repeated, count only the first time used, but continue to count any novel portion of the sentence (e.g., "Pues . . . ," "Bueno . . . ," "Es que . . . . ").

8. Echolalic reproductions by the child of the adult's utterance are not counted, but if the utterance is changed in any way, it is counted.

9. Sentences that contain English words are omitted.

10. Rules for scoring. Each category is given specific points depending on the level of complexity. See Table 5–12 for the Spanish scoring system. Table 5–13 is DASG analysis form.

   a. Indefinite pronouns and noun modifiers receive points.

   b. Pronouns must agree in number with the corresponding verbs.

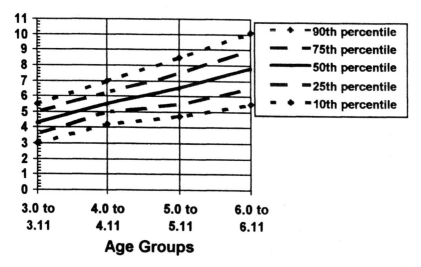

Figure 5–1. Percentiles for Average Scores of 128 Mexican-American and Puerto Rican Children. (From "Developmental Assessment of Spanish Grammar," by A. S. Toronto, 1976. *Journal of Speech and Hearing Disorders, 41,* p. 164. Copyright 1976 by the American Speech-Language-Hearing Association. Reprinted with permission.)

    c. A noun modifier must agree in number and gender with the noun it modifies.

    d. "una" and "la" are not counted when used as articles.

    e. Plural indefinite pronouns or noun modifiers are given a score of four (or more).

11. Computing the average score (AS). The individual scores for each sentence are added together and divided by the total number of sentences scored. This provides a mean score which is the average score (AS). This score is compared to the DASG norms to estimate the child's grammatical proficiency.

B. Categories

1. Personal pronouns

    a. Includes personal, relative, and reflexive pronouns.

    b. Person, number, gender, and case must be correct to allot credit.

Table 5–12. Syntactic Hierarchies and Scoring System for the Developmental Assessment of Spanish Hrammar (DASG)

Score	Indefinite Pronouns and Noun Modifiers	Personal Pronouns	Primary Verbs
1		*Reflexives:* se, me, te	*single present tense:* vengo, vienes, viene. *Copular* es, son, esta, estas estar + V + ndo with *present tense only:* esta jugando.
2	este, esta, esto, ese esa, eso	*1st and 2nd person singular:* yo, tu, Ud., mi, mio, tuyo, suyo, su.	*plural conjugations, preterit tense, imperatives—any form*
3	la, lo mas, todo, toda otro, otra, nada, primero	*3rd person:* el, ella, de, el, de ella, alguien, aquel *singular direct object and indirect object:* se, me, te, le, ti *also:* conmigo, contigo	*copula other than score 1:* fue, era, fui past perfect tense: -aba and ia endings *subjunctives*
4	*all plurals up to and including this level:* algo, alguno, alguna, poco, mucho, unos, uno, dos, tres	*plurals:* nosotros, nuestro, ellos, ellas, Uds., mis, tus, sus, aquellos, tuyos, suyos, nadie	
5	cualquier, ambos, cada, ningun	*plural direct object and indirect object:* les, los, nos	poder or deber + V + r *conditional tense:* podia, estaria
6			haber + V + do
7	varios, unico, proximo, ultimo, segundo, tercero, etc. *plus female genders*	*relative pronouns:* que, quien, cual	haber + estado + V + ndo
8			poder or deber + haber + estado + ndo *passives*

continued

Table 5–12. Syntactic Hierarchies and Scoring System for the Developmental Assessment of Spanish Grammar (DASG) *(continued)*

Score	Secondary Verbs	Conjunctions	Interrogative Words
1			qué quién dónde
2	*Complementing infinitives:* ir + infinitive Va a salir. Iba a venir Dejale cantar. Me gusta caminar. Tiene que ir.		cuándo para qué cómo
3	*Present participle:* Va llorando. Anda buscando.		por qué de quién de qué cúanto(s)
4	*Noncomplementing infinitives of purpose:* Se pararon a jugar. para salir, de venir. *Also infinitive with interrogative word:* Se donde ir.	y que	cúal
5		porque para que como pero, cuando	
6		donde, entonces, mientras, hasta, antes, desde, despues, aun, menos que	
7	*Passive complement of infinitve:* Quiero estar ni vestido.	o si	
8	*Gerund or infinitive used as subject:* Fumar es malo. Caminando le hace bien.	por lo tanto, sin embargo, no obstante sino, etc.	

Table 5–13. Developmental Assessment of Spanish Grammar

Name: _____   Date: _____

Birth Date: _____   C.A.: _____

Examiner: _____

No. of sentences in sample: _____

Total points: _____

D.A.S.G. Score: _____

Sentences	Indefinite Pronouns	Personal Pronouns	Primary Verbs	Secondary Verbs	Conjunctions	Interrogative Words	Total

Page _____ of _____

c. Indefinite pronouns used as personal pronouns are scored as indefinite pronouns, (e.g., "lo" and "la").

d. The pronouns "se," "me," and "te" must be identified as either reflexive pronouns or indirect objects:
(1) Reflexive: The pronoun is part of the verb action and is directed toward the subject of the sentence: (e.g., "se fue el," "se baño ella").
(2) Indirect object: The pronoun is the recipient of the action described by the verb (e.g., "me gusta," "se lo dio").

2. Primary verbs

Schema for primary verb conjugation:

a. PN = person and number. Determines verb ending (first person singular third person plural).

b. T = time, mood, aspect. Determines verb tense (present, past, subjunctive, conditional).

c. PN + T + (poder + r/deber + r) (haber + do) (estar + ndo) V.

d. Poder/deber = modal auxiliary verbs used with infinitive form of another verb ("Yo puedo venir." "El debe pagar.").

e. Haber = auxiliary verb used with past participle form of a verb ("Yo podría haber venido." "Yo he venido.").

f. Estar = auxiliary verb used with present participle form of another verb ("Yo estoy viniendo.") *Note:* Estar can be used as an auxiliary verb or a copula and must be differentiated during analysis; for example, auxiliary: "El esta corriendo"; copula: "El esta aquí."

g. Infinitive verbs other than those noted in the schema are analyzed as secondary verbs.

h. Production.
(1) Errors due to poor articulation are scored as correct.
(2) Incorrect production of the following verbs are scored as correct as long as all other parts of the verb are correctly

used in the sentence: "qauero" for "quiero," "tene" for "tiene," "vene" for "viene."

i. Incorrect conjugation of a verb does not receive a score.

3. Secondary verbs

When two kernel sentences are combined by making the second verb an infinitive, present participle, or gerund, a secondary verb is formed. Examples of secondary verbs follow.

a. Complementing infinitives = infinitives which complete a secondary thought of a primary verb.
   (1) ir + a + infinitive (va a dormir.)
   (2) querer + infinitive (quiero caminar.)
   (3) saber + infinitive (el sabe manejar.)
   (4) dejar + infinitive (dejale salir.)
   (5) gustar + infinitive (me gusta comer.)
   (6) tener + que + infinitive (tiene que salir.)
   (7) *Note:* The obligatory "a" after "ir" and the "que" after "tener" must be present for the secondary verb to be scored.

b. Present participles of the secondary verb are used in conjunction with a primary verb in the form of a present participle (-ndo). When used with the verb "estar," it is counted as part of the primary verb. Example: Va llorando. Anda buscando.

c. Noncomplementing infinitives of purpose = infinitives which are attached to existing complete sentences and are preceded by a preposition. Example: Se pararon *a jugar.* Se pusieron los abrigos *para salir.*

d. Infinitives occurring after interrogative words (e.g., "se donde ir").

e. Passive complement of infinitive (e.g., "Quiero estar vestido").

f. Gerund or infinitives used as subjects (e.g., "fumar es malo").

4. Conjunctions

a. Sentences that begin with conjunctions are counted as complete sentences, but the conjunction is not scored (e.g., "(y) Maria va a comer.").

b. Only one "y" conjunction per sentence is allowed when it connects two independent clauses. Sentences are broken up as:
(1) "Yo tengo un perro y me hermano tiene un gato."
(2) "(Y) a mi mama no le gustan y dice que no los quiere en la casa."

c. When "y" is used in a series or in a compound subject or predicate, it is always counted and does not require the sentence to be broken up (e.g., "A mi me gustan galletas y dulces y tortillas y helado.").

d. Internal conjunctions other than "y" do not require the sentence to be broken up (e.g., "el quería salir pero estaba lloviendo y no tenía abrigo.").

e. Overused conjunctions are not counted (e.g., "entonces" el perro lo comio entonces el niño se enojo").

5. Interrogative words are scored when used in a question. Care must be taken to distinguish between interrogative words and conjunctions.

VII. CONCLUSION

This chapter provided guidance in a few experimental procedures for the analysis of Spanish form. The analysis of form has been neglected over the years in the assessment of Spanish-speaking children. This is probably because of the limited number of Spanish-speaking speech-language pathologists. Limiting a language analysis to use only limits the diagnosis of the language impairment to one area of language. A thorough analysis of a language sample must include form, content, and use from samples collected for Spanish-speaking children.

CHAPTER

6

Intervention

The ultimate goal we have for each client is to provide an intervention program that meets the individual's needs. There are numerous language development programs that focus on either the form, content, or use of language. The selection of one of these areas for therapy will depend on the severity and needs of each client. This chapter does not review or suggest any particular program for therapy with Spanish-speaking children. Instead, this chapter reviews aspects that are important for the provision of services to Hispanic children. These include models for speech and language services, variables that influence the selection of the language of instruction, teaching and learning strategies known to be effective with second-language learners, characteristics of Hispanic children that will affect the interactions within therapy sessions, suggestions for therapy in language and phonology, adaptation of materials to be culturally and linguistically sensitive to Hispanic students, and suggestions for parent involvement.

I. MODELS FOR SPEECH AND LANGUAGE SERVICES

Bilingual special education uses three basic models for providing services to special needs children. A fourth combined model is used in large school districts. These models are described in terms of speech-language pathology and the culturally and linguistically diverse student population.

A. Bilingual Support Model

The monolingual speech-language pathologist is the main service provider, but uses a technician or speech-language assistant who is bilingual to provide the service in the minority language. The assistant may act as the interpreter for the speech language-pathologist or be an independent assistant whose therapy is programmed by the clinician.

B. Coordinated Service Model

This is a bilingual team approach with a monolingual speech-language pathologist and a bilingual speech-language pathologist. Both work to provide services to students, the former in English and the latter in the minority language. The bilingual clinician provides services to predominately Spanish-speaking children, the monolingual speech-language pathologist is the primary service provider in the school building.

C. Integrated Bilingual Model

The primary service provider is the bilingual speech-language pathologist. This person is responsible for all intervention programs for the Hispanic student in both languages.

D. Combination of the Bilingual Support and Coordinated Models

A monolingual speech-language pathologist and a bilingual assistant provide services in English and Spanish, with the professional assistance and guidance of an itinerant bilingual speech-language pathologist who develops programs in Spanish for several assistants in the large school system.

II. ALTERNATIVE STRATEGIES FROM ASHA (1985)

A. Establish Contacts

Bilingual speech-language pathologists can be hired as consultants to provide assessments and treatment to minority-language students.

B. Establish Cooperative Groups

A group of school districts or programs might hire an itinerant bilingual speech-language pathologist to provide services for a specific language group.

C. Establish Networks

University and work settings could develop ties so that minority professionals can be recruited into the workforce.

D. Establish Clinical Fellowship Year and Graduate Practica Sites

Graduate students from bilingual communicative disorders programs could be supervised by bilingual speech-language pathologists and assist personnel in schools as assistants in assessment and intervention of language-minority students.

E. Establish Interdisciplinary Teams

A team approach can be implemented to include the monolingual speech-language pathologist with bilingual professionals from other fields, such as psychology, to provide assessment of language minority students.

III. CLINICIAN'S ROLE

A. An active role must be taken by the speech-language pathologist in the treatment of bilingual or monolingual Spanish-speaking children whether the clinician is monolingual or bilingual (Kayser, 1993). The areas of focus for treatment may include:

1. Counseling of Family

a. The rights of the client should be relayed to the parents. They must be informed of the child's legal rights for services. Also, the parent must be informed of the child's potential and skills that can be developed through intervention. The parents' beliefs from and experiences in another country may influence their understanding of intervention and the child's development.

b. Future bilingualism. The clinician must encourage the use of Spanish in the home. The exclusion of the home language from intervention is detrimental to a child's cognitive development. Therefore, the following hypotheses may be given as reasons for the maintenance of the home language and its use to assist the child.

(1) **Threshold hypotheses** (Cummins, 1984) proposes a minimum level of linguistic competence which a child must attain in order to avoid cognitive deficits. If there is a low competence in L1 it is likely that a similar low level will be present in L2. Parents should provide sufficient maintenance and support for the home language in order to obtain a similar level of competency in the second language.

(2) **Developmental interdependence hypothesis** (Cummins, 1984) assumes that if the outside environment provides sufficient stimuli for maintenance of L1, then intensive exposure to L2 in the school leads to rapid bilingual development with no detrimental effects to the first language.

(a) If the child is in an English-only classroom, the parents can be instructed to provide the child's language needs in the home language.

(b) The parents' involvement with language intervention becomes critical to the development of English and cognition.

c. Parents' role in language development

(1) Language use within typical Hispanic homes varies from typical mainstream homes. Conversation and narratives.

(a) Discussion of home rules with the parents and the clinician's explanations of what is expected from children in school will help parents understand that there is more to language than simply talking more to their child.

(b) Rules on how greetings are accomplished, who may start a conversation, what topics may be discussed, what is tolerated in taboo words during conversations, and what is appropriate for differing age groups are all important areas of discussion with the family.

(2) Open versus closed family systems (Heath, 1989): Parents should be made aware that a child's exposure to different language usage comes from interaction with people from outside the family and the community. The mainstream

norms for requesting, asking questions, using politeness formulas, and asking for clarifications are all possible language usages a child should be exposed to and should learn. Parents must be counseled to understand that withholding interactions with mainstream communities limits opportunity in English language learning for a child.

(a) Open families allow their children to have contact with the mainstream community.

(b) Closed families prefer to maintain the traditional values and means of interactions.

2. Coordinating services with other professionals (i.e., ESL, bilingual education, special education) is another area of support in treatment that the speech-language pathologist may develop.

   a. A group of professionals may work with a bilingual student, each having a specific goal.

   b. The speech-language pathologist coordinates the services.

   c. Data from all of the specialists working with the second language learner are compiled to determine a child's progress and determine future team goals.

B. Determining the Language of Intervention

1. There is no set rule for determining which language should be used for intervention (N. Miller, 1984).

2. A number of factors that should be considered from Ortiz (1984) are listed. Included below are my (H. K.) comments about these factors.

   a. **Client/parent preference.** [Although the parent may prefer English, the parent should be counseled to allow the home language as the language of intervention.]

   b. **Age of student.** [Younger students should have the home language as the language of instruction. Older students may need more assistance with English].

   c. **Type and severity of communication disorder.** [Any child with any type of disorder may benefit from therapy in the home language.]

d. Availability of bilingual personnel. [The single most influential reason for providing services in English could well be that there are not enough professionals who can provide speech and language services in the native language.]

e. Length of residency. [The longer that the child has been in the United States, the more likely that the child will receive therapy in English. The reasoning may be that the child, with time, may lose the ability to speak the home language.]

f. Motivation for learning English. [Children with little motivation to learn English would probably best be served in the home language. Those who do not want to maintain Spanish may benefit from combined English and Spanish therapy.]

g. Attitude toward mainstream culture. [If the child's and family's attitude is positive, English therapy may be beneficial. If not, Spanish should be targeted.]

h. Intellectual abilities. [This may not have as much influence on which language should be targeted, because intellectual abilities may not be an important criterion for learning a second language.]

i. Language aptitude. [This may be an important variable as to which language should be the language of intervention, but not enough is known about this area and its impact on language learning in students with language impairments.]

j. Progress in therapy. [This has to be assessed on an individual basis. Lack of progress may not result from the language of instruction, but the language of instruction may interact with other variables that influence a lack of progress.]

3. The optimal language of instruction depends on the child's relative language proficiency is the premise of Langdon and Saenz (1995).

  a. If a language-disordered child is strongly dominant in English, provide intervention in the stronger language.

  b. If a language-disordered child is strongly dominant in the native language, provide intervention in the native language.

    c. If a bilingual language-disordered child has somewhat stronger skills in the native language, the clinician should consider providing bilingual services.

4. There is specific support for intervention in the native language from a number of sources.

    a. For a child to benefit fully from instruction in a second language, his or her skills must be developed to a threshold in the first language (Cummins, 1984; Perozzi & Sanchez, 1992).

    b. What is learned in the native language will transfer to a second language.

    c. Children with normal language skills often develop stronger English proficiency when they are taught bilingually.

    d. Research in speech-language pathology supports the hypothesis that the native language may be instrumental in helping minority-language children with language impairments to develop skills in both the native and the majority language (Kiernan & Swisher, 1990; Perozzi, 1985; Perozzi & Sanchez, 1992).

    e. Experimental single-subject designs by Perozzi (1985) and Kiernan and Swisher (1990) support the use of the first language before instruction in the second language and suggest that a bilingual curriculum is better than teaching only in English.

IV. DETERMINING INTERVENTION GOALS

Miller (1984) suggests:

A. The core content of remediation for the person who is bilingual does not need to differ from that used with monolingual children.

B. The clinician should treat only those aspects that impair intelligibility and not dialect or the influence of the first language on English.

C. Therapy in English should begin with features of language that the child commands in the first language and that have identical or nearly identical structural characteristics in both languages.

V. CHARACTERISTICS OF A TYPICAL HISPANIC CHILD'S SOCIALIZATION AND ITS APPLICATION TO INTERVENTION

A. Planning (Delgado-Gaitan, 1987)

Planning by Hispanics generally is accomplished within a group and not individually. It's believed that the wisdom of the group allows for better decisions. Therapy adaptation to socialization would mean that decisions about session objectives and in what sequence these are presented could be determined by the group of children in treatment.

B. Work Style (Delgado-Gaitan, 1987)

Hispanic work style is cooperative. That is, Hispanic children will work together to accomplish a goal, but each will contribute what is believed to be his or her best or preferred task. A therapy rework would mean that cooperative learning may be more effective with Hispanic children than competitive work assignments.

C. Time Orientation (Kayser, 1995a)

Hispanic groups have been described as polychronic in time orientation. Tasks may not be completed in a linear manner (monochronic). Therapy adaptation would mean that time allotted to specific activities or objectives would be determined by the interest level of the children. What may be of interest to the group may be worked on several times during a therapy session.

D. Interaction

Heath (1986) and Harry (1992) describe Hispanic children as preferring peer-peer interactions rather than adult-child interactions. Clinical application would mean that these children would probably benefit more from group therapy than individual therapy in which the interaction would be child-child adult-child.

E. Field-Dependent or -Sensitive (Ramirez & Castañeda (1974)

Individuals have been described as having certain personal and learning characteristics. All Hispanic children do not have these characteristics, but these should be considered when providing intervention. These children may have a tendency to display the following characteristics:

1. Like to work with others to achieve a common goal;

2. Like to assist others;

3. Are sensitive to feelings and opinions of others;

4. Openly express positive feelings for the teacher;

5. Ask questions about the teacher's tastes and personal experiences;

6. Seek guidance and demonstration from the teacher;

7. Seek rewards that strengthen a relationship with the teacher;

8. Are highly motivated when working individually with the teacher;

9. Prefer performance objectives and global aspects of the curriculum to be carefully explained;

10. Prefer to have concepts presented in humanized, or story format; and

11. Prefer to have concepts related to personal interests and experiences.

VI. EFFECTIVE TEACHING STRATEGIES FOR HISPANIC STUDENTS

Beaumont (1992) reports that effective teaching emphasizes the whole instead of the parts and focus on language use rather than form, alone. Effective teaching requires:

A. Authentic, purposeful communication interactions to teach language skills;

B. Activities that use whole texts, themes, events, and experiences;

C. Incorporating children's home/community communication events into activities;

D. Connecting intervention activities to a larger curriculum context;

E. Creating an environment conducive to a wide range of language uses;

F. Integrating form, content, and use in activities; and

G. Planning intervention around a vision of effective communication and learning rather than around deficits.

VII. COGNITIVE LEARNING STRATEGIES

Chamot and O'Malley (1986) recommend cognitive learning strategies as part of the intervention for Hispanic students. They provide students with strategies to help students learn language through the use of language. The following are some suggestions.

A. Resourcing: Using reference materials, such as glossaries, dictionaries, encyclopedias, and information available in textbooks. Learning to enlist other people to assist in locating and determining information.

B. Transforming: Changing the form of a word, phrase, or sentence grammatically.

C. Grouping: Classifying words, terminology, or concepts according to their attributes and semantic categories.

D. Note Taking: Writing down key words and concepts in an abbreviated form during a listening or reading activity.

E. Deducing: Applying rules to understand or produce language or solve problems.

F. **Imagining:** Using visual images in understanding and remembering new information

G. **Elaborating:** Linking new information to what is already known or providing a story grammar that incorporates the new information in meaningful ways.

H. **Transferring:** Using what is already known to facilitate a new learning task, and linking new information with what is already known.

I. **Inferencing:** Using context clues to guess meanings of new items, predict outcomes, or fill in missing formation.

VIII. SOCIAL AND AFFECTIVE LEARNING STRATEGIES

Chamot and O'Malley (1986) found that other strategies can also be part of the learning of language for second language learners. The following are some strategies.

A. **Questioning:** Learning to elicit from a teacher or peer explanation, clarification, and rephrasing of examples.

B. **Cooperation:** Learning to work with peers to solve a problem, pool information, check a learning task, or get feedback on oral or written performance.

C. **Self-talk or Other Assisted Talk:** Reducing anxiety by using mental techniques for one to feel competent to accomplish a task; practicing and talking through tasks.

D. **Modeling:** Learning to observe and imitate others' performance in the process of learning and performing.

IX. METACOGNITIVE LEARNING STRATEGIES

Chamot and O'Malley (1986) found that the following strategies will assist the student in academic assignments and achievement.

A. Advance Organizers: Previewing the main ideas and concepts of material to be learned.

B. Selective Attention: Attending to key words, phrases, sentences, or other specific types of information.

C. Organizational Planning: Planning the parts, sequence, and main ideas to be expressed.

D. Self-Monitoring: Checking comprehension during listening or reading or checking the accuracy and appropriateness of one's oral or written production while one speaks or writes.

E. Self-Evaluation: Deciding how well one has accomplished a learning activity.

X. MONITORING AND ADAPTING YOUR SPEECH TO SECOND-LANGUAGE LEARNERS

The teacher/clinician should assist the second language learner during therapy interactions by self-monitoring and adapting speech used for instruction (Zehler, 1994). The use of examples is an important strategy that speech-language pathologists may use as part of therapy. The following are suggestions.

A. Restate complex sentences as a sequence of simple sentences.

B. Avoid or explain use of idiomatic expressions.

C. Restate at a slower rate when needed, but with typical intonation and stress patterns.

D. Pause often to allow students to process what they hear.

E. Provide specific explanations of key words and special or technical vocabulary.

F. Provide explanations for the indirect use of language.

G. **Introduce objects, photographs,** or other materials as examples.

H. **Use visual organizers and graphics** to organize and illustrate key points.

I. **Use demonstrations or role playing** to illustrate concepts.

J. **Provide notes or an outline of the lesson** for later review by students.

K. **Allow time for students to discuss** what they learn and to generate questions that require clarification.

XI. INSIGHTS INTO U.S. CHILDREN'S ENGLISH-AS-A-SECOND-LANGUAGE (ESL) READING

R. B. Barrera (1997) provides a summary of the literature concerning literacy for second language learners.

A. Reader Background Characteristics

ESL readers reflect diverse backgrounds and experiences (different native languages, native-language literacy levels, years of schooling, ages of entry into the United States, and so forth) which influence second-language reading in varying ways.

B. Comparison of L2 Reading and L1 Reading

In terms of basic cognitive processes, second-language reading appears to be more similar to native-language reading than different. Differences occur in the amount of use and length of time accorded to certain processes. For example, in comparison to native-language readers, advanced- and intermediate-level ESL readers tend to read and to monitor comprehension more slowly, use fewer and some different metacognitive strategies, and recall subordinate ideas less well (J. Fitzgerald, 1995).

C. Role of Home Language and Home Culture in L2 Reading

Children's home language and culture are resources for developing second language reading proficiency.

1. Readers transfer native language knowledge to ESL reading and often demonstrate second-language comprehension more effectively in their native language than in English. Use of the home language and incorporation of the home culture into school's curriculum and instruction should be encouraged (J. Crawford, 1997; Cummins, 1981; Cummins, 1996).

2. Children who develop first-language knowledge and skills fully during the preschool years often make the transition to schooling in English more easily and effectively than children who do not maintain the home language. However, more research is needed on the early emergence and development of ESL reading in preschool and elementary school students (J. D. Ramirez, Yuen, Ramey, Pasta, & Billings, 1991).

D. Relationship Between L2 Orality and L2 Literacy

The existing research is unclear on the relationship between ESL reading proficiency and ESL oral proficiency. The notion that English orality must be developed to an optimal level for English literacy to develop merits further and more refined examination. In some cases, second-language speech, reading, and writing appear to develop simultaneously (J. Fitzgerald, 1995).

E. ESL Instruction Practice

The more sources of information that beginning second-language readers have from which to construct meaning, the better.

1. Teachers of second-language learners need an expansive repertoire of strategies for making abstract skills and concepts across the curriculum concrete and meaningful for ESL readers. Because language (and second-language literacy) are acquired more effectively when they are learned in conjunction with meaningful content and purposeful communication, language and content learning in ESL instruction should be combined (C. J. Ovando & Collier, 1998; Peregoy & Boyle, 1993; Berhnardt & Kamil, 1998).

2. Texts that are comprehensible, interesting, and meaningful are essential for reading to, with, and by ESL readers. Culturally familiar texts may be especially helpful, because prior knowledge of story elements may make the stories more comprehensible than unfamiliar texts. It is desirable that ESL learners be read to on a daily basis

by individuals who are fluent models of skilled English reading (S. Hudleson, 1994).

3. Learning a second language (including second-language literacy) is not an end in itself, but a means to achieving social integration and academic success. Teachers should facilitate the integration of second-language students with native-English-speaking students and unify the curriculum for all learners, making necessary adaptations to render material more accessible to and equitable for ESL learners. Second-language learners need to confront cognitively challenging content that goes beyond mere rote material and results in the application of critical thinking (F. Genesee, 1994).

4. To promote the comprehension and participation of ESL students, second-language reading instruction should provide individual attention; small-group interaction; and other shared, collaborative activities. Less fluent/proficient readers might be paired with more fluent peers some of the time (D. Johnson, 1994).

F. Teacher Knowledge

Teachers must know the backgrounds of their ESL students to plan effective instruction for them and conduct valid assessments of youngsters learning and literacy (F. Genesee & Hamayan, 1994).

XII. SUGGESTIONS FOR HELPING A CHILD TO READ

Literacy is central to the learning of a second language. Four areas for particular focus are word recognition, language competence, strategies for reading, and using familiar frameworks (Sutton, 1989). Suggestions are:

A. Word Recognition

1. Label items, locations, and activities in the room.

2. Write directions, schedules, calendar information, names, and work duties on the chalkboard.

3. Use language experience activities to describe events in the classroom.

4. Include simple reading/writing activities for beginning-level students as reinforcement for language practiced orally.

5. Write down familiar dialogues and stories and practice these as choral reading, role playing, and so on.

6. Have students search and identify words in printed material that they would like to know.

7. Provide students with a place to keep track of important words, for example, a notebook.

B. Language Competence

1. Describe familiar values expressed in stories, folklore, maxims, and historical tales.

2. Introduce unfamiliar vocabulary.

3. Conduct prereading discussion of concepts important to understanding a particular selection.

4. Provide group assignments, allowing students to work with others to process the text and discuss the ideas.

5. Monitor students' comprehension by questioning them and having students talk about what they have read in their own words.

C. Strategies

1. Help students establish a personal rationale for reading to direct their attention to the task.

2. Familiarize students with the language of different types of reading materials, for example, stories, science text, drama, and so on.

3. Incorporate learning strategies such as taking notes, integrating new information into an existing knowledge framework, and making word associations.

4. Demonstrate scanning, skimming, reading for main idea, and reading for details.

5. Introduce summarizing, self-monitoring, recalling events in chronological order, retelling in one's own words, outlining, and use of graphic organizers.

D. Familiar Frameworks

1. Use folk tales and stories from the students' native culture.

2. Employ materials with familiar experiences and characters.

XIII. DEFINING WHOLE LANGUAGE

Whole language is a philosophy or attitude about how people learn; not a program or a curriculum. It applies to all ages and not just children. It reflects the ways we learn beyond school as well as in school. It helps students learn to speak, read, and write well in a wide variety of situations (Goodman, Goodman & Flores, 1979; Holdaway, 1979).

A. Whole language is reading, writing, thinking, and speaking that crosses the curriculum and is student-centered and dynamic.

B. Assumptions About Whole Language

1. **Emergent literacy skills.** The individual has an awareness that symbols relate meaning.

2. **Book handling skills.** The child has knowledge about the use of a book and how it is used.

3. **Metalinguistic awareness.** The individual can think about reading.

C. Whole Language Methods That Promote Reading in a Second Language

1. **Language experience approach** (Goodman et al., 1979). Based on the idea that children are better able to read materials from their own experiences and oral language. It involves eliciting oral language from the children and then shaping their language into written material.

2. **Shared Reading** (Holdaway, 1979). The beginning reading experience is through big books with high interest stories in large print. The children participate through listening, choral reading, or individual reading.

3. **Sustained silent reading.** The children and teacher are involved in silent reading.

4. **Dictated stories.** Group writing of a story.

5. **Creative writing.** Children learn to write about any topic of interest.

6. **Dialogue journal writing.** Children write personal notes and entries into a notebook that the teacher reads and then writes responses.

D. Other Opportunities for Writing

1. **Daily schedule.** Writing date, written daily schedule, signing up for activities.

2. **Functional communication.** Making lists such as supply lists; writing teacher or parent reminder notes; developing memo board for oneself, other students, school activities, asking questions; having a complaint box; taking notes by telephone for the school office or nurse; practicing writing name, address, and phone number.

3. **Self-expression and interpersonal communication.** Writing journals, stories about selected pictures; stories about newspaper articles; describing a friend, toy, animal or object; writing how-to descriptions; writing notes and letters to friends, relatives, classmates; writing about feelings and happenings, plans for future, books read; planning charts for self and group.

XIV. ACTIVITIES FOR ORAL LANGUAGE DEVELOPMENT

It is important to use these activities in both languages.

A. Poetry: This can be presented in each language, but also poetry using code switching may be displayed and taught.

B. **Finger Plays**

C. **Mother Goose rhymes** and other rhymes from the home culture

D. **Puppets** (stick, sack, felt, cone, sock, glove, finger)

E. **Telephone:** A telephone is not always a common object in Hispanic homes. Therefore, some children may not know telephone scripts, for example, the sequence of the greeting, asking for a desired individual, and so on. Moreover, many Hispanic children may be taught that the telephone is not a toy and children do not play with it.

F. **Conversation:** Encourage it during art activities.

G. **Props:** Clothing, such as hats, doctor outfits, mail carrier uniforms, and so on.

H. **Objects:** Show different objects and ask children how many different names they can think of for them, employing such props.

I. **Recordings:** original poems or songs that the children can comment on.

J. **Stories:** Discuss a story and allow the children to retell, using visual aids, a wordless book, group retelling, or explaining to each other.

K. **Television:** Make a large cardboard TV set and slide pictures into the window and ask children to tell about them.

L. **Naming:** The teacher points to a body part and children name it, or the teacher shows an object or picture and they name it.

M. **Field Trip:** Discuss preparations, such as what children should ask, what they think they will see, and how they should act.

N. **Boxes:** Put a number of textured objects in a box with small holes for the children to reach into and feel and describe the objects.

O. Songs: The Hispanic culture is rich with songs that are taught in schools and in the home. This is a valuable resource for language development.

P. Questions: Ask open-ended questions that require thought and verbalization rather than (close-ended) yes, no, or one-word answers; propose questions (why, what, where, when, how) and assist the children in finding the answers.

Q. Tape Recorder: Have pupils speak into it and listen to the playback.

R. Videotape: Let the children view a the tape with sound level at zero and supply the dialogue.

S. Definitions: Introduce new terms and provide an opportunity for the children to practice giving their meanings.

T. Food Experiences: Let the children help shop, prepare, and eat different foods.

U. Dramatic Play: Provide an area in the room where children can reenact community themes, for example, fire fighting, hairstyling, camping, and so on.

V. Lessons in Cause-and-Effect: Show pictures and discuss situations, asking, "What would happen if?"

W. Show and Tell: Hispanic children may not have learned this type of narrative, therefore, provide opportunities for children to develop it.

X. Spotlight: Place a display and rotate the contents weekly. Give children enough time to enjoy and investigate the contents.

Y. Microphone: Encourage children to pretend they are talking through a microphone.

XV. INTERVENTION FOR PHONOLOGY

The literature in phonology and emergent literacy indicates that phonological awareness is important in the development of reading abilities. This is an important area of development for the Spanish-speaking preschooler, who will likely be presented with English literacy without first being introduced to reading in the native language. Because Spanish phonology is a simpler system than English, it is paramount that children have a sound, intact Spanish phonological system as they acquire English language skills.

A. Issues in Treating Phonological Disorders
(Goldstein, 1995).

1. A phonological analysis should be completed in both languages.

2. No studies yet indicate when it is appropriate to conduct therapy for phonological disorders in Spanish and when therapy should be in English.

3. Effectiveness of therapy techniques has not been addressed.

B. Selecting Phonological Targets for Beginning Cycles
(Mann & Hodson, 1992)

1. Begin with early developing patterns such as stops, nasals, glides, and labials.

2. Word-final singleton consonants can be developed at a later time, eventually for English.

3. Posterior/anterior consonant contrasts.

4. Children who demonstrate backing need to learn to produce alveolar consonants and hear contrasts between alveolars and velars.

5. Early targeting of /s/ plus stop consonant sequences is inappropriate for Spanish-speaking children. Use a technique that emphasizes and prolongs the vowel following a strident.

6. /l/ and /r/: target these at the end of each cycle, because Spanish-speaking children with normal phonological development produce these by age 5 years.

7. Consonant sequences should be produced in their entirety.

8. All remaining consonant sequences, multisyllabicity, and complex consonant sequences should be the focus of therapy.

9. The clinician should assess the child's vocabulary by prompting for names of common objects to determine the unfamiliarity of words used in therapy.

XVI. INTERVENTION FOR NARRATIVES

The production of narratives in the school setting is critical for academic success (Gutierrez-Clellan, 1995). But, we know that narrative development and production will vary from culture to culture. Children who are identified with a language impairment may benefit from direct instruction in school-related narratives. Parent participation for this type of intervention in the native language will help the child learn to produce narratives that are expected in the school setting.

A. Parents Have an Influence on the Child's Use of Narratives

B. Recommendations for Parents (Gutierrez-Clellan, 1995)

1. Do not ask too many questions or questions unrelated to your child's own version of a past event. The questioning will disrupt the child's attempts at producing a coherent narrative.

2. Requests for clarification or informative expansion may be more helpful in eliciting children's narrative productions than requests for overt productions.

3. Topic switching may not be a useful strategy in promotion of the child's narrative learning.

4. Stimulate a child's narrative ability by prompting the youngster to relate novel past events.

5. Prompting for unshared experience (experience only of child) has been found to be more helpful than prompts for shared experiences (family experiences).

6. Participant variances can also be due to the type of narrative being told: cuentos (folktales), family cuentos (stories about a wayward uncle), and personal past experience (how the family immigrated to the area).

7. Use "dile" in interactions with three people to teach and practice descriptions of daily routines and events.

XVII. GENERAL CONSIDERATIONS ON ADAPTATION

Typically, speech-language pathologists have been most concerned with culturally and linguistically appropriate assessment. The intervention process has not been well addressed within speech-language pathology. Commercially available materials have been developed with themes that are familiar to typical mainstream homes. These materials need to be adapted to serve the needs of children who have speech and language impairments and who come from a diverse background. The following are general guidelines in adapting materials (Hoover & Collier, 1989).

A. Use a committee to assess the appropriateness of adapted materials.

B. Document the success of selected materials.

C. Adapt only specific materials requiring modifications and do not attempt to change too much at one time.

D. Try out different materials and adapt until you have achieved an appropriate education level for each student.

E. Strategically implement material adaptation to ensure smooth transition into new materials.

F. Follow a consistent format or guide when evaluating materials.

G. Follow a well-developed process for evaluating the success of adapted or developed materials.

XVIII. ADAPTATION FOR THE SPECIAL NEEDS STUDENT

A. The first step is to compare the characteristics of the material or techniques with the characteristics of the learner in three different areas (Cheney, 1989):

1. The achievement level of the student and the instructional level of the material

2. The learning characteristics of the student and the modes of presentation response required by the material or instructional technique

3. The motivational characteristics of the student and the motivational qualities of the material

B. Once these areas have been compared, some adaptations that can be made are (Hoover & Collier, 1989).

1. Adjust method of presentation or content

2. Tape record directions for the material

3. Provide alternative methods for responding to questions

4. Rewrite brief sections to lower the reading level

5. Outline material for the student before reading a selection

6. Reduce the number of pages or items on a page to be completed by a student

7. Break tasks into similar subtasks

8. Provide additional practice time to ensure mastery

9. Substitute a similar, less complex task for an assignment deemed as too demanding.

XIX. ADAPTATION OF MATERIALS FOR CULTURAL APPROPRIATENESS

Commercial materials may be used with Hispanic populations, but these typically are not culturally appropriate. These materials may not reflect the typical life environments for many Hispanic students and may convey stereotypes for a number of culturally and linguistically diverse groups (see Appendix F). The following are suggestions for adapting materials (Carrasquillo, 1992)

A. Check for stereotypes and biases in materials representing the cultures of Hispanics. Some concepts/issues that teachers have identified as presenting Hispanics in a stereotyped or biased format in educational materials are:

1. Time—the notion that time or punctuality are not important elements of daily life

2. Machoism—this stereotype includes assigning an animal nature to Hispanic males (complementary domains of authority)

3. Hispanics as shy/passive individuals, portrayed in secondary/menial roles

4. Having low self-image

5. All Hispanics as people of color

6. Disadvantaged

7. Lower intelligence

8. Parental role in education as uninvolved

9. Language limited—the idea that all Hispanics speak Spanish or are not proficient in English

10. Sexism—Hispanics are assigned social or professional roles depending on their gender

B. Check the content of and tasks requested by the materials (Collier & Kalk, 1989; Kayser, 1989).

1. If knowledge is typical of home, school, preschool

2. Do tasks appear unnatural for Hispanic members of the reviewing committee?

3. Appropriateness of vocabulary for community use and familiarity by children

4. Committee reactions to picture stimuli for cultural accuracy of picture representation

5. Familiarity of story content for area (urban vs. rural) with topics, objects, animals, and so on that are seen and spoken about within the community.

6. Does the child have the necessary preskills for the task?

7. Do the materials contradict the child's cultural beliefs? If the contradiction is unavoidable, then discuss both sides and represent the two beliefs as different.

8. Will the material require using competitive or cooperative rewards in the lessons?

C. Look at storytelling and everyday experiences of the community (Kayser, 1989).

1. Attempt to develop storytelling for the community. What is told? How is it told.

2. What is valued in good storytelling? Who can tell stories? What is bad storytelling?

3. Use stories familiar to Hispanic children by questioning parents.

4. Change pictures and objects as necessary to depict the experiences of children of the community.

D. Do an assessment of adapted materials with a committee of a speech-language pathologist, bilingual specialist, psychologist, special education teacher, and a bilingual community member (Kayser, 1989).

E. Try to include some of the following aspects into the materials (Collier & Kalk, 1989).

1. The diversity of the Hispanic community: not all Hispanics have the same characteristics.

2. The shared identity among Hispanic communities: language and backgrounds.

3. A realistic representation of the community: educational, economic, political characteristics.

4. Contemporary life experiences: urban and rural.

5. Language accuracy: standard Spanish and dialectal variation for the region.

XX. BUILDING BRIDGES BETWEEN PARENTS AND SCHOOL

An important aspect of intervention is the involvement of parents. The following are variables to be considered when developing parent programs in the schools.

A. Many recently arrived Mexican families see the school as the sole authority on what needs to be learned and how it should be done (Scarcella, 1990).

B. Parents teach their children to be respectful to elders and to care for their own actions, but they rarely work with their children on school-related activities (Delgado- Gaitan, 1987).

C. The reasons that many Hispanic parents are less involved in school-related activities than English-speaking parents has as much to do with the school's unfamiliarity with non-English-speaking communities as it does with these communities' unfamiliarity with the schools (Faltis, 1995).

D. General announcements and invitations to parents in the language of the home need to be written 1 week before an event, with a short reminder the day before.

E. Send information on what to expect in meetings and provide a purpose and activity schedule.

F. Encourage other families in other classrooms to talk among themselves about meetings and school events.

G. Even if the parent is illiterate in Spanish, Hakuta (1990) has shown that bilingual children from third grade on are capable of translating English to their native language and vise versa.

H. **Immigrant parents may have** little understanding about how U.S. schools work, and parents may not believe that schools prepare all children equally (Torres-Guzman, 1995).

I. **Parents may get involved,** if their child's teacher reaches out to them and gives them multiple opportunities to become involved at home and in school.

J. **There needs to be a balance** between a teacher learning about a child's home environment and the parent learning about the school environment.

XXI. CONCLUSION

Providing appropriate intervention services will require more than the traditional approach of individual or group treatment twice a week. Collaboration with other professionals in the school environment is necessary. A number of variables have been discussed that should be considered in the intervention process. The most important of these is the cooperation of parents in the development of the child's bilingualism and the incorporation of the native language in literacy. Both of these areas, although out of the scope the hands-on intervention of the speech-language pathologist, are important for the long-term well-being and the academic success of Hispanic children who are functioning in two languages and two cultures.

APPENDIX

A

Raising a Bilingual Child

ADVANTAGES

- Bilingual persons can communicate with a wider variety of people than monolingual persons.

- Bilingual persons can experience two or more cultures.

- Bilingual persons can build bridges to an extended family who speak the ancestral language, helping to create a sense of belonging and rootedness to the family and culture.

- Bilingual persons may have an economic advantage as businesses become more multinational, requiring the services of individuals who can speak multiple languages and have knowledge of various cultures.

IMPORTANT FACTORS

- Make language learning fun and enjoyable; do not stress correctness of grammar.

- Encourage use of the minority language; provide opportunities for using the minority language for meaningful communication.

KNOWING IF LANGUAGE DEVELOPMENT IN EACH LANGUAGE IS NORMAL

- Each child's language development varies and is dependent on the amount of exposure to each language.
- Normal language developmental patterns:
  1 year—First understandable words
  2 years —Two-word combinations, increasing to three- and four-word combinations
  3 years —Increasingly longer sentences that reflect normal grammar
  4 years —Increasingly more complex sentences

IMPACT OF SECOND LANGUAGE ON FIRST LANGUAGE

- Bilingual persons may develop more sensitivity and awareness to languages and the needs of listeners.
- Bilingual persons have multiple pathways for accessing information stored in the brain.
- Knowledge developed in one language can be accessed through a second language once the vocabulary has been learned. The concepts do not have to be retaught in the second language.
- Children may initially mix words from both languages, but the interference is temporary.
- Children may not have as large of a vocabulary as a monolingual person, but the combined number of words from the two vocabulary systems is greater than that of a monolingual individual.

IMPACT OF BILINGUALISM ON INTELLIGENCE

- Bilingual persons who have equal abilities in both languages are found to have slightly higher IQ scores than monolingual persons.
- Bilingual persons tend to be more flexible, fluent, and original in their responses to open-ended type questions than monolingual persons.

- Bilingual persons' increased awareness of language (metalinguistic skills) aids in earlier development of literacy skills.

IMPACT OF BILINGUALISM ON THINKING SKILLS

- Bilingual children have a wider set of associations for vocabulary, which allows them to look at an issue or problem with more options for problem solving or comprehensive understanding.
- Bilingual children may be more conscious of language and more sensitive to the needs of listeners.

IMPACT OF BILINGUALISM ON THE FUNCTION OF THE BRAIN

- Bilingual persons seem to process and store information in the brain in the same manner as monolingual individuals.
- There is no evidence that bilingualism harms the functioning of the brain.

IMPACT OF BILINGUALISM ON FUTURE SUCCESS

- Bilingual persons will have better employment prospects and economic success.
- Bilingual individuals may have improved social success through increased cultural sensitivity leading to enhanced interpersonal skills.
- Bilingual persons will gain political success by having skills in both native and majority languages.

EFFECT ON CHILDREN BEING TRANSLATORS/INTERPRETERS

- Children may gain positive self-esteem and develop a closer relationship to their families when translating from majority to native language for parents.
- Children may be strained by the advanced language used in an adult conversation or by the emotional or private nature of information being translated.
- Children might be expected to "show-off" their translation skills.

IMPACT OF BILINGUALISM ON CULTURAL IDENTIFY

- There are three basic types of cultural identity seen in bilingual persons.

  1. Bicultural—the bilingual individual is able to switch easily between two cultures.
  2. Minority culture rootedness—the bilingual person firmly maintains roots in the minority culture.
  3. Dislocation—the bilingual individual no longer has roots to the minority culture and has not developed a connection to the majority culture.

- The bilingual child should be given experiences in the minority culture to offset the overabundance of experiences he or she will be exposed to in the majority culture.

EFFECT OF BILINGUALISM ON SOCIAL DEVELOPMENT

- Bilingual persons tend to have an advantage in social relationships. They are able to interact with a wider variety of people and develop more diverse friendships than those who speak only one language.

- There may be prejudice of minority language speakers by majority language users. Teachers and parents should help to facilitate understanding and acceptance of differences by all children.

BILINGUALISM AND LEARNING DIFFICULTIES

- Bilingualism is rarely the cause of learning difficulties. Language-based learning difficulties can occur when neither language is sufficiently developed for the child to succeed in the school curriculum.

- Even children who learn at a slower pace can develop skills in two languages.

BILINGUALISM AND EMOTIONAL/BEHAVIORAL PROBLEMS

- Bilingualism does not cause emotional or behavioral problems. Being part of a social group which is undervalued or discriminated against by the majority culture can create emotional or behavioral problems, but bilingualism is not the cause of the problem.

SHOULD TWO LANGUAGES CONTINUE TO BE USED WITH CHILDREN WITH DIAGNOSED LANGUAGE DISORDERS OR EMOTIONAL PROBLEMS?

- Try to determine the cause of the problem. Rarely is it caused by bilingualism.

- Changing from bilingualism to monolingualism may worsen a problem. An immediate change in the home environment might cause emotional stress exacerbating the situation.

- If a change to monolingualism is required by the nature of the problem, the child's home language should be retained. Once the diagnosed problems have been remediated, bilingualism can be reintroduced.

DOES BILINGUALISM CAUSE STUTTERING?

- There is no evidence that stuttering is caused by bilingualism.

- If a parent is anxious about a child's language development, this anxiety may be passed to the child, making language learning an unenjoyable experience.

SHOULD I FOLLOW THE ADVICE OF PROFESSIONALS WHO TELL ME TO RAISE MY CHILDREN MONOLINGUALLY?

- Many times the professionals who offer this advice are monolingual individuals who are not educated in bilingualism.

- Current research indicates that the positive benefits of raising bilingual children outweigh the negative.

WILL A CHILD'S PERFORMANCE IN SCHOOL BE AFFECTED BY BILINGUALISM?

- If the child is expected to learn in a language that is underdeveloped or below the level demanded in the curriculum, the child will be at a disadvantage.

- Undervaluing of bilingualism by the majority culture may reduce the bilingual child's self-esteem and confidence in his or her learning abilities.

SHOULD MY CHILD BE PLACED IN A BILINGUAL
SPECIAL EDUCATION PROGRAM?

- Ensure that the child has been correctly diagnosed as having a disorder. At times, the testing materials used to identify disorders are based on the majority language, therefore a test might well not accurately reflect the capabilities of a child using a minority language.

- If the child has been properly diagnosed with a disorder, then the child will benefit from a bilingual special education program, rather than a monolingual program.

WHAT IS THE FUTURE OF BILINGUALISM
IN THE GLOBAL ECONOMY?

- There will continue to be a need for people to act as interpreters and translators in the global economy.

- As the divisions between countries continue to become less well-defined, many people are returning to their cultural roots, including the languages that support those cultures.

Source: Adapted from *A Parents' and Teachers' Guide to Bilingualism* by C. Baker, 1995. Clevedon: Multilingual Matters Ltd.

A P P E N D I X

B

Criando a un hijo Bilingüe

VENTAJAS

C Las personas bilingües se pueden comunicar con una variedad más amplia de personas que las personas monolingües.

C Las personas bilingües tienen la oportunidad de conocer dos culturas o más.

C Las personas bilingües pueden crear puentes entre la familia extendida que hablan un idioma ancestral así ayudando a pertenecer y ser parte de las raíces de la familia y cultura.

C Las personas bilingües pueden tener ventajas economicas, puesto que ahora en día, muchos negocios se están desarrollando con un enfoque más internacional que requiere de los servicios de individuos que pueden hablar idiomas múltiples y que tienen el conocimiento de varias culturas.

FACTORES IMPORTANTES

C Procure que el aprendizaje del lenguaje se disfrute y sea divertido; no ponga un énfasis a la exactitud de la gramática.

C Fomente el uso del idioma materno; proporcione oportunidades para usar el idioma materno en actividades significantes comunicativas.

EL DESARROLLO NORMAL EN CUALQUIER IDIOMA

C Todo desarrollo del lenguaje varía y es dependiente de la cantidad de exposición a cada idioma.

C Aprendiendo dos idiomas puede ser un proceso más lento que el aprender un idioma. Pero las etapas del desarrollo son iguales en cada idioma.

C El patrón de desarrollo normal del lenguaje:
1er año—Primeras palabras reconocibles
2do año—Combinaciones de dos palabras, que se incrementa a combinaciones de tres y cuatro palabras
3er año—Oraciones más largas que reflejan la gramática normal
4to año—Incrementando a oraciones más complejas, cada vez más.

EL IMPACTO DE UN SEGUNDO IDIOMA EN EL PRIMERO

C El conocimiento desarrollado en un idioma puede ser conocido en el segundo idioma, una vez que se haya aprendido el vocabulario en el idioma materno. Los conceptos no tienen que volverse a enseñar en el segundo idioma.

C Inicialmente los niños intercambiarán palabras de los dos idiomas, pero esta interferencia es temporal.

C Niños posiblemente no tengan un vocabulario tan extenso como los niños monolingües, sin embargo, la combinación de número de palabras de los dos vocabularios es mayor que esos de un niño monolingüe.

EL IMPACTO DEL BILINGÜISMO EN LA INTELIGENCIA

C Las personas bilingües que tienen habilidades iguales en los dos idiomas, se han encontrado por tener coeficientes intelectuales (IQ) más altos que personas monolingües.

C Las personas bilingües tienden a ser más flexibles, creativos y demuestran mayor fluidez en sus respuestas a preguntas con respuestas amplias que personas monolingües.

C La incrementada conciencia de lenguaje (habilidades metalinguisticas) que poseen las personas bilingües, ayuda en el desarrollo más temprana de habilidades literarias.

EL IMPACTO DEL BILINGÜISMO EN HABILIDADES DE RAZONAMIENTO

C Los niños bilingües tienen un vocabulario más amplio para hacer asociaciones que les permite ver un problema o cuestiones con más opciones para resolver problemas o para tener un entendimiento comprensivo.

C Los niños bilingües posiblemente sean más concientes sensibles a las necesidades del oyente.

EL IMPACTO DEL BILINGÜISMO EN LAS FUNCIONES DEL CEREBRO

C Las personas bilingües aparentemente procesan y guardan información en el cerebro en la misma manera que los monolingües.

C No hay evidencia que el bilingüismo tiene efectos negativos en el funcionamiento del cerebro.

EL IMPACTO DEL BILINGÜISMO EN EL EXITO FUTURO

C Las personas bilingües tendrán un prospecto mayor para ser empleados y de exito económico.

C Las personas bilingües posiblemente tengan mayor éxito social a través de un aumento de sensibilidad cultural que de tal manera mejora las habilidades interpersonales.

C Las personas bilingües obtendran éxito politico a traves de sus habilidades en su idioma materno y de la sociedad de mayoria.

LOS EFECTOS DE LA TRADUCCION E INTERPRETACION EN EL NIÑO

C Los niños posiblemente obtengan una mejor auto estima y desarrollarán una relación más cercana a su familia cuando traducen del segundo idioma a su idioma materno para sus padres.

C Posiblemente los niños se sientan agobiados por tratar de traducir el idioma avanzado usado por los adultos o por la naturaleza de cuestiones emocionales o privados de la informacíon que se les pide que se traduzca.

EL IMPACTO DEL BILINGÜISMO EN LA IDENTIDAD CULTURAL

C Se han encontrado tres identidades culturales en personas bilingües:

1. Bicultural: la persona bilingüe puede cambiar fácilmente entre las dos culturas.
2. Raíces en la cultura minoritaria: la familia bilingüe mantiene sus raíces en la cultura minoritaria.
3. Dislocación: la persona bilingüe no tiene raíces en su cultura minoritaria y no ha desarrollado una conexión con la cultura mayoritaria.

C Al niño bilingüe se le debería de proporcionar oportunidades en la cultura minoritaria para balancear la cantidad de experiencias que van a tener con la cultura mayoritaria.

EL EFECTO DEL BILINGÜISMO EN EL DESARROLLO SOCIAL

C Las personas bilingües tienden a tener una ventaja en las relaciones sociales. Tienen la capacidad de interactuar con una variedad más amplia de personas y para desarrollar amistades diversas.

C Prejucios ante personas que hablan un segundo idioma por la cultura mayoritaria puede suceder. Maestros y padres deberían de ayudar a facilitar la comprensión y la aceptación de las diferencias entre las dos culturas.

EL BILINGÜISMO Y DIFICULTADES DEL APRENDIZAJE

C Raramente el bilinguismo es causa de problemas del aprendizaje. Problemas basados en el lenguaje pueden suceder cuando ninguno de los dos idiomas se ha desarrollado suficientemente para tener éxito con el curriculum escolar.

C Aún niños que aprenden a un paso más lento, pueden desarrollar habilidades en los dos idiomas.

EL BILINGÜISMO Y PROBLEMAS EMOCIONALES Y DE CONDUCTA

C El bilingüismo no causa problemas emocionales y de conducta. Perteneciendo a un grupo social la cual es devaluada o es discriminada por la cultura mayoritaria puede crear problemas emocionales y de conducta, pero ser bilingüe no es la causa del problema.

SE DEBERÍA DE SEGUIR USANDO DOS IDIOMAS CON NIÑOS QUE TENGAN UN PROBLEMA DIAGNOSTICADO EN LENGUAJE O PROBLEMAS EMOCIONALES?

C Trate de determinar cual es la causa del problema. Raramente es causado por el hecho de ser bilingüe.

C Cambiando de ser bilingüe a monolingüe puede agraviar el problema. Un cambio radical en el ambiente de la casa puede causar estres emocional, agraviando más la situación.

C Si un cambio a ser monolingüe es necesario por la naturaleza del problema del niño, el idioma materno del niño debería ser mantenido. Una vez que los problemas diagnosticados han sido remediados, el bilingüismo se puede reintroducir.

CAUSA TARTAMUDES EL BILINGÜISMO?

C No hay evidencia que el bilingüismo causa tartamudes.

C Si un padre está ansioso del desarrollo del lenguaje de su hijo, esta anciedad puede ser pasado al niño, haciendo que el aprendizaje del lenguaje ya no sea una experiencia que se disfrute.

DEBERIA DE TOMAR LOS CONSEJOS DE LOS PROFESION-ALES QUE ME DICEN QUE CRIE A MIS HIJOS COMO MONOLINGÜES?

C Muchas veces los profesionales que ofrecen estas recomendaciones son monolingües que no han recibido educación en temas sobre el bilingüismo.

C Las investigaciones presentes indican que los beneficios positivos de criar hijos bilingues son mayores a las consecuencias negativas.

SERA AFECTADO EL RENDIMIENTO ESCOLAR DE UN NINO POR SER BILINGÜE?

C Si a un niño se le espera que aprenda en un idioma subdesarrollado o si las expectativas son menores a la demanda del curriculum escolar, el niño si estará en desventaja.

C La devaluación del ser bilingüe por la cultura mayoritaria puede reducir la auto estima y confianza del niño bilingüe en sus habilidades para aprender.

EL EFECTO DE LA INSTRUCCION DEL IDIOMA MATERNO EN EL DESARROLLO DEL IDIOMA MAYORITARIO

C Normalmente a los niños instruidos en su idioma materno, han tenido amplias oportunidades para desarrollar el idioma mayoritario. Mucho cuidado se debería de proporcionar para que se les expongan amplias oportunidades en el idioma mayoritario a niveles academicos avanzados.

DEBERIA DE PARTICIPAR MI HIJO EN UN PROGRAMA DE EDUCACION ESPECIAL BILINGÜE?

C Asegurese que su hijo ha sido evaluado correctamente, y que realmente tenga un problema. En ocaciones las pruebas que se usan para hacer las evaluaciones y para identificar problemas son basados en el idioma mayoritario, por lo cual las pruebas no reflejan las capacidades actuales de un niño usando su idioma materno.

C Si el niño ha sido diagnosticado con un problema, correctamente, entonces si tendría beneficios en el participar en un programa de educación especial bilingüe, en vez de un programa monolingüe.

CUAL ES EL FUTURO DEL BILINGÜISMO EN LA ECONOMIA GLOBAL?

C Seguira habiendo una necesidad para personas que actuen como interpretes y traductores en la economia global.

C Mientras que las divisiones entre países continuen a ser menos definidas, mucha gente está regresando a sus raíces culturales, incluyendo a los idiomas que apoyan estas culturas.

A P P E N D I X

C

Examines de Apraxia Oral

Presente cada orden dos veces como mandato verbal y una vez en imitación para todos los pacientes. Califique cada respuesta. Para el primer intento diga, "Voy a pedir que haga algunas cosas con su lengua y boca escuche bien y haga exactamente lo que pido" Para el segundo intento diga, "Bueno, tratamos otra vez." Para imitación diga, "Bueno, ahora míreme bien y haga exactamente lo que hago.

	Intento 1	Intento 2	Intento 3
1. Abra su boca.			
2. Saque su lengua.			
3. Muéstreme/enséñame como se sopla.			
4. Muéstreme/enséñame sus dientes.			
5. Haga sus labios redondos.			
6. Trate de tocar su nariz con su lengua.			

7. Muerda su labio inferior/bajo. _____ _____ _____

8. Lama sus labios en un círculo. _____ _____ _____

9. Saque su lengua algunas veces. _____ _____ _____

10. Muéstreme/enséñame como tirita. _____ _____ _____

11. Muéstreme/enséñame como se sonríe. _____ _____ _____

12. Muéstreme/enséñame como claquear
su lengua. _____ _____ _____

13. Muéstreme/enséñame como besaría
un bebe. _____ _____ _____

14. Trate de tocar su quijada con su lengua. _____ _____ _____

15. Llene sus mejillas con aire. _____ _____ _____

Examin Para la Apraxia del Habla

Indicaciones generales "voy a pedir que diga algunos sonidos, palabras y oraciones.
Escuche bien y repita exactamente lo que digo. Está listo? "Diga estos sonidos y
manténgalos en mayor tiempo posible."

                             Intento 1   Intento 2   Intento 3

1. Diga /a/ y manténgala el mayor tiempo
posible. _____ _____ _____
2. Diga /i/ y manténgala el mayor tiempo
posible. _____ _____ _____
3. Diga /o/ y manténgala el mayor tiempo
posible. _____ _____ _____

"Ahora quiero que diga otros sonidos. Esta vez dígalos lo más rápido que pueda."

4. Diga /pʌ pʌ pʌ pʌ pʌ pʌ/ _____ _____ _____

5. Diga /tʌ tʌ tʌ tʌ tʌ tʌ tʌ tʌ/ _____ _____ _____

6. Diga /kʌ kʌ kʌ kʌ kʌ kʌ / _____ _____ _____

7. Ahora diga los tres sonidos juntos, como esto.
/pʌtʌkʌ, pʌtʌkʌ, pʌtʌ kʌ/ _____ _____ _____

	Intento 1	**Intento 2**	**Intento 3**

Ahora quiero que diga algunas palabras después de que yo las digo."

	Intento 1	Intento 2	Intento 3
8. televisión	___	___	___
9. bicicleta	___	___	___
10. escalera	___	___	___
11. elefante	___	___	___
12. Ningaturtle	___	___	___
13. zoológico	___	___	___

"Diga estas palabras después de que yo las diga."

	Intento 1	Intento 2	Intento 3
14. mas	___	___	___
15. masa	___	___	___
16. masaje	___	___	___
17. que	___	___	___
18. querido	___	___	___
19. queso	___	___	___
20. pan	___	___	___
21. pana	___	___	___
22. panela	___	___	___
23. sol	___	___	___
24. sola	___	___	___
25. solaso	___	___	___

	Intento 1	Intento 2	Intento 3

"Diga estas palabras después de que yo las diga."

26. mamá

27. chancho

28. papá

29. sillas

30. coco

31. dedo

32. lila

33. rara

34. bebé

35. galgo

"Repita estas oraciones después de yo."

36. Por favor ponga las compras en la refrigeradora.

37. Arturo era un hombre gordo y feliz.

38. En verano venden vegetales.

39. El reloj costoso está perdido.

40. Juan comió pan y café.

Calificación General

Indique la presencia o ausencia de las siguientes características de la apraxia del habla.

	Presente	Ausente

1. Errores foneticas predominantes
   • más sustituciones que omisiones y distorciones
   • adiciones
   • repeticiones

2. Errores preservatorios y anticipatorios

3. Los errores son aproximaciones de la producción deseable

4. Busca la posición articulatoria correcta

5. Los errores son muy inconsistentes

6. Los errores aumentan cuando el tamaño de las palabras aumenta

7. Hay periodos de producción sin error

8. Hay menos errores en el habla automatica

9. Respuestas en imitación son podres

10. El paciente reconoce sus errores pero no puede anticiparlos ni corregirles

11. Desórdenes prosódicos
    velocidad lenta

    acento normal

    espacio entre palabras igual

A P P E N D I X

D

Spanish Case History Form
Historia de Habla y Lenguaje

IDENTIFICACION:

Nombre: _____ Fecha de nacimiento: _____

Domicilio _____
        calle   cuidad   estado   z.p.

Número de teléfono _____ Sexo _____ Edad _____

Referido por _____ Médico _____

DESCRIPCION DEL PROBLEMA:
Describa el problema del habla o lenguaje del niño (a) _____
_____
_____

En su conocimiento, cuando se dio Ud. cuenta del problema? _____

_____

_____

HISTORIA DE LA FAMILIA:

	Nombres	Edad	Ocupacíon	Educacíon

Madre: _____

Padre: _____

Niños: _____

Otras personas:

_____

_____

Que idioma(s) se habla en el hogar? _____

DURANTE EL EMBARAZO DE ESTE NINO (A) HUBO:

toxemia (envenenamiento de la sangre) _____

Diferencia entre los tipos de sangre _____

Diabetes _____

Sarampíon Aleman _____

Enfermedades (mencione especificamente) _____

_____

Golpes o heridas (mencione especificamente) _____

_____

Medicacíon _____

radiografías (rayos X) _____

Hemorragías _____

Anemia _____

Otros _____

_____

Fue este niño (a) prematuro?

Favor de indicar como fue este parto:

Normal _____

De operacíon cesarea _____

Venia de pies _____

Otros _____

Sufrio complicaciones en el embarazo? _____

_____

Durante el primer mes su niño (a) tuvo . . .?

Falta de oxigeno _____

piel amarilla _____

que pasar tiempo en la incubadora _____

    Por cuanto tiempo? _____

Problema al mamar or al comer _____

Babeaba demasiado _____

DESARROLLO:
Escriba el edad cuando su niño/(a) . . :

se sentó solo _____

gateo _____

se paró solo _____

caminó solo _____

tuvo contról del orín _____

Hubo algo en el desarrollo de su niño (a) que le preocupo durante los primeros 18 meses?

HISTORIAL MEDICO:
Enfermedades previas. (Favor de indicar la fecha y la edad del niño (a) cuando tuvo estas enfermedades, se es qúe las padecio).

Sarampíon _____

Encefalitis _____

Meningítis _____

Viruela loca (varicela) _____

Paperas _____

Fracturas en los brazos o en las piernas _____

Fracturas en el craneo (descalabradas) _____

Contuciones (golpes) _____

Ingestíon de veneno (tomo veneno) _____

Infecciones continuas en los oidos _____

Infeccíon respiratoria _____

Pulmonía _____

Alergías _____

Otros _____

Describa las veces que fue hospitalizado, incluyendo las visitas a la sala de emergencia. Cual fue la razon de las visitas y la fecha? _____

_____

Describa la salud de su niño (a). _____

_____

Tiene su niño?:

Defecto visual _____ Usa lentes? _____

Defecto del oído? _____ Usa aparato para oír? _____

Abertura en el paladar? _____

Defecto en la lengua, quijada, dientes, labios? _____

Problemas emocionales o del comportamiento? _____

_____

Defecto fisico? _____

HABLA Y LENGUAJE:
Hizo su niño (a) sonidos durante los primeros seis meses? _____

Que edad tenía cuando hablo su primera palabra? _____

Que edad tenía cuando empezó a usar dos o tres palabras combinadas? _____

Por lo regular, cuantas palabras usa en frase hoy? _____

COMPRENSION: Indique si o no

    Entiende solamente movimientos expresivos _____

    Responde a mandatos simples o sencillos _____

    Responde a mandatos verbales complicados _____

EXPRESION:

    Se comunica principalmente por medio de acciones _____

    Conversa con frases simples _____

    Habla con palabras limitadas o frases sencillas _____

    Conversa a un nivel normal o avanzado _____

HABLA:

    Se da a entender solamente con los padres o familiares _____

    Se da a entender con otras personas _____

FLUIDEZ:

    Normal _____

    Repite palabras _____

    Repite silabas _____

    Repite sonidos _____

    Prolonga sonidos _____

    Tension en la cara _____

Comprende (reconoce) su niño (a) que tiene problemas con el habla? Si la respuesta es afirmativa, Cuando se dio cuenta? _____

_____

Ha tratado de corregirse a si mismo? _____
Como lo ha hecho? _____

Presenta este niño (a) algun problema de comportamiento?

    en casa _____

en el barrio o vecinidad _____

en la escuela _____

HISTORIA EDUCATIVA:
Escriba el nombre de las escuelas a las que haya asistido, incluyendo las escuelas pre-escolares.

Escuela	Ciudad	Fecha	grado o año

RESUMEN:
Si ud. fuera la persona que evaluara los factores que podrían estar relacionados con los problemas de habla y lenguaje de su niño (a), que más agregaría?
Marque los factores que Ud. cree que exístan.

Problemas del oído _____ Problemas al tomar alimento _____

Problemas emocionales _____ Falta de amigos con quien jugar _____

Parálisis cerebral _____ Falta de estímulo adecuado _____

Epilépsia _____ Problemas de comportamiento _____

Disturbio visual

Celos hacia los hermanos _____ Problemas del ambiente _____

Caprichudo (terco) _____

_____

Nombre de la persona quien llenó esta forma

_____   _____

Fecha   Cual es su relacíon familiar con el/la niño (a)

Source: St. Mary's Hospital & Health Center, Tucson, Arizona, Texas Christian University, Fort Worth, Texas. Adapted by H. Kayser, 1994.

A P P E N D I X

E

Spanish/English Preschool Screening Test
Hortencia Kayser, Ph.D.

Name: _____   Date: _____

Age: _____   Date of Birth: _____

Teacher: _____   Clinician: _____

Accept a response in either English or Spanish.

I. Identifying Information

1. Cómo te llamas? What is your name?
2. Cómo se llama tu mamá/papá/hermano/hermana?
   What is your mom's/dad's/brother's/sister's name?
3. Cuántos años tienes? How old are you?

II. Body Parts

The child is asked to name each of the 12 body parts listed below. If child does not name, then ask child to point to the body part. *Enseñame tu* _____. *Dónde está tu* _____? Show me your _____. Or where is your eye?

1. el ojo (eye)
2. la boca (mouth)
3. el diente (tooth)
4. la mano (hand)
5. el pie/accept pata (foot)
6. el oído/la oreja (ear)
7. la nariz (nose)
8. la pierna (leg)
9. el brazo (arm)
10. el cuello/pescueso (neck)
11. el dedo (finger)
12. la espalda (back)

III. Describe Noun Functions

The child is asked to give the primary function for each of the nouns below. The following practice items may be presented to demonstrate the task:

Para qué se usa la cama? What is a bed used for? If the child does not talk, ask the child to show you what it is used for.

Item   Response

1. escoba (broom)
   Para qué se usa la escoba?
   (Enseñame/show)

2. Peine (comb)
   Para qué se usa el peine?
   (Enseñame/show)

3. Pelota (ball)
   Para qué se usa la pelota?
   (Enseñame/show)

4. vaso (glass)
    Para qué se usa el vaso?
    (Enséñame/show)

5. comida (food)
    Para qué se usa la comida?
    (Enséñame/show)

6. cama (bed)
    Para qué se usa la cama?
    (Enséñame/show)

7. silla (chair)
    Para qué se usa la silla?
    (Enséñame/show)

IV. Basic Spatial Concepts

Haz lo que te digo. Do what I tell you to do.

| Instruction | Response |

1. Pon las manos detrás de tu cabeza.
    Put your hands behind/in back of your head.

2. Pon las manos debajo de la mesa.
    Put your hand under the table.

3. Párate en frente de la silla.
    Stand in front of the chair.

4. Párate a un lado de la silla.
    Stand beside the chair.

5. Pon el (carro, zapato, pelota) adentro de la caja.
    Put the (car, shoe, ball) inside the box.

6. Pon la cuchara en la taza.
    Put the spoon in the cup.

V. Imitation of Sentences. (Spanish Only)

1. Son pollos (Present indicative, 2 years)

2. Está alla.

3. Yo tengo zapatitos (N+V+DO) (3 years)

4. La agarró esta muchachita. (preterit, 3 years)

5. Caminaba así. (imperfect indicative, 3 years)

6. Comí yo blanquillos/huevos. (V+S+DO)

7. Me está pintando los zapatos. (present perfect indicative, 3–4 years)

8. Yo no he ido al circo. (present perfect indicative, 3–4 years)

9. Perdío la llanta el bos. (V+DO+S, 4 years)

10. Te dije que lo hicieras así. (present subjunctive, 3–4 years)

Imitation of Sentences. (English Only)

1. The car is going. (2 years)

2. This is mine. (2 years)

3. I like ice cream.

4. He wanted to come too. (3 years)

5. Mommy said I can't go.

6. My mommy and I went to the store. (4 years)

7. My daddy drove me to school. (4 years)

8. Jerry ran to the swing.

9. We were going swimming. (5 years)

10. I will clean my room tomorrow. (5 years)

VI. Imitation of Sequencing pattern

The clinician knocks the pattern on the table. *Haz esto.* Do this.

Example	Response

1. X
2. XXX
3. XX
4. XXXX
5. XXX
6. XXXXX

VII. Following Instructions

1 step—Tócate la nariz.

2 step—Dame el carro y el zapato.

3 step—Abre el libro; levanta la mano, dame el carro.

4 step—Párate, abre la puerta, siéntate, y levanta la mano.

VIII. Articulation:

Test: _____

Raw Score: _____

Intelligiblilty: _____

Comments:

Subtest Raw Scores: **Pass/Fail**

   I.   /3

   II.   /12

   III.   /7

   IV.   /6

V.   Spanish   /10   English   /10

VI.   /6

VII.   /4

Total   /48

A 3 year old child should be able to achieve a score of 30 or above.
A 4 year old child should be able to achieve a score of 38 or above.

A P P E N D I X

F

Resource List

FAMILY RESOURCES

Spanish

1. APUNTES PARA LA FAMILIA
   http://www.aacap.org/apntsfam/index.htm

2. DISFONIAS INFANTILES
   www.sinfomed.com/luis.txt

3. DESARROLLO DE LOS RECIEN NACIDOS
   www.exnet.iastate.edu/pages/nncc/ChildDev/sp.des.rec.nac.html

4. REPERCUSION EMOCIONAL DEL NINO CON LABIO Y PALADAR HENDIDO
   ourworld.compuserve.com/homepages/ROBERTO_MURGUIA/la-pa-hen.htm

5. MI PEDIATRIA-INFORMACION RELACIONADA CON LA SALUD DE LOS NINOS
   www.mipediatria.com.mx

6. EL NINO QUE TARTAMUDEA EN LA ESCUELA
www.stuttersfa.org/br_spnts.htm

7. PUERTO RICO STATE RESOURCE
www.ldonline.org/finding_help/local_org/puerto_rico.html

8. PUERTO RICO RESOURCES-NATIONAL INFORMATION CENTER FOR CHILDREN AND YOUTH WITH DISABILITIES
www.nichey.org/stateshe/pr.htm

9. PREGUNTALE A NOAH SOBRE LA SALUD PERSONAL
www.noah.cuny.edu:8080/sp/wellness/healthyliving/spersonalhealth.html

10. PAGINA DE ANDRES SAUCA LINGUISTICA Y LOGOPEDO (INFORMACION, ENVIAR E-MAIL CON PREGUNTAS)
www.ctv.es/USERS/asauca/home.html

English (provides good information to families)

1. KIDSOURCE ONLINE
www.kidsource.com

2. KIDSEARS-THE HEARING AND LANGUAGE DEVELOPMENT RESOURCE
www.kidsears.com

3. SMILES-A GROUP OF DEDICATED FAMILIES WHO HAVE DEVELOPED A FIRST-HAND UNDERSTANDING OF THE NEEDS OF CHILDREN WITH CLEFT LIP, CLEFT PALATE, AND CRANIOFACIAL DEFORMITIES.
www.cleft.org

4. WIDESMILES: CLEFT LIP AND PALATE RESOURCE
www.widesmiles.org

5. APRAXIA-KIDS
avenza.com/~apraxia/index.html

SPEECH-LANGUAGE PATHOLOGIST'S RESOURCES

1. SERVICIO DE LOGOPEDIA
www.vanaga.es/barajas/Logo.htm

2. LOGOPEDIA: GENERALIDADES SOBRE LA REHABILITACION DE LA VOZ (TEMAS DE LOS TRASTORNOS DE LA VOZ)
www.centreorl.net/temas/

3. LOGOPEDIA ONLINE
   www.filnet.es/freeusersofilnet/logopedia/LOGOPEDI2.HTM

4. CENTER FOR THE STUDY OF AUTISM (VISION GLOBAL DEL AUTISMO)
   www.autism.org/translations/spanish.html

5. CENTER FOR MULTICULTURAL RESOURCES
   Utexas.edu/coc/csd/multicultural/index.html

6. Bilingual education Resources on the Internet
   http://www.edb.utexas.edu/coe/depts/ci/bilingue/resrouces.htmi

7. Bilingual Education Resources on the Net
   http://www.estrellita.com/%7Ekarenm/bil.htmi

8. Bilingualism and Languages Network
   http://giraffe.rmpic.co.uk/orgs/bln

9. Office of Bilingual Education and Minority Languages Affairs
   http://www.ed.gov/pubs/TeachersGuide/pt16.html

10. Curriculum Networking Specialists
    hhtp://www.he.net/~epc

11. Center for the study of books in Spanish for children and adolescents
    hhtp://www.scusm.edu/campus_centers/csb/index.htm

12. BEN: Bilingual/ESL Network
    http://tism.bevc.blacksburg.va.us/BEN.html

13. U.S. Department of Education
    http://www.ed.gov/index/html

14. Bilingual Book Consultants
    http://tism.bevc.blacksburg.va.us/EMAC/emac.html

15. Internet Resources for Bilingual Education and ESL
    http://scholastic.com/el/exclusive/links1095.html

16. National Clearinghouse for Bilingual Education
    http://www.ncbe.gwu.edu/. . ./

17. Bilingual Research Center
    http://zzyx.usc.edu/Cntr/brc.html

PUBLISHERS FOR READING AND MATERIALS IN SPANISH

Publishers

Continental Book Company
625 E. 70th Ave. #5
Denver, CO 80229
1-303-289-1761

Miller Educational Materials, Inc.
ESL Catalog
7300 Artesia Blvd.
Buena Park, CA 90621
1-800-636-4375

Addison-Wesley
ESLI Bilingual Catalog
1 Jacob Way
Reading, MA 01867-9984
1-800-552-2259

Bilingual Education Service, Inc.
Children's Literature in Spanish
2514 South Grand Ave.
Los Angeles, CA 90007-9979
1-800-448-6032

Barron's Education Series, Inc.
250 Wireless Blvd.
Hauppauge, NY 11788
1-800-645-3476 Ext. 204, 214, or 215

National Textbook Co.
ESL and Bilingual Education
4255 East Touly Ave.
Lincoln Wood, IL 60646-1975

TESTS AVAILABLE IN SPANISH

Assessment of Phonological Processes
Los Amigos Research Associates
7035 Galewood
San Diego, CA 92120
(619) 286-3162
Tests articulation in single words and focuses on analyzing phonological
    processes.
Ages 3;0 years and above

Austin Spanish Articulation Test
DLM Teaching Resources
One DLM Park
Allen, TX 75002
Tests articulation in single words.
Ages 3;6–12;0 years

Del Rio Language Screening Test
National Educational Laboratory
P.O. Box 1003

Austin, TX 78767
Tests receptive vocabulary, oral commands, sentence repetition, and story
    comprehension.
Ages 3;0–6;0 years

Medida Espanola de Articulacion (MEDA)
San Ysidro School District
2250 Smyth Ave
San Ysidro, CA 92173
Tests articulation in single words.
Ages 4;0–9;0

Preschool Language Scale—3 (PLS-3)
Psychological Corporation
Harcourt Brace & Company
555 Academic Court
San Antonio, TX 78204
1-800-228-0752
Tests language comprehension and production.
Ages birth–6;11 years

Pruebas de Expresion Oral y Percepcion de la Lengua Espanola (PEOPLE)
Los Angeles County Office
9300 E. Imperial Highway
Downey, CA 90242
Tests memory, auditory association, sentence repetition, story comprehension, and
    encoding.
Ages 6;0–9;11 years

Screening Test of Spanish Grammar (STSG)
Northwestern University Press
1735 Benson Ave
Evanston, IL 60201
Tests receptive and expressive structures.
Ages 3;0–6;6 years

Spanish Articulation Measures
Academic Communication Associates
Publication Center, Dept. 206
4149 Avenida de la Plata
P.O. Box 586249
Oceanside, CA 92058
(619) 758-9593

Tests phonological processes through repetition, stimulability, spontaneous word production, and conversation.
Ages 3;0 years and above

Structured Photographic Elicitation Language Test **(SPELT) (two levels)**
P.O. Box 12
Sandwich, IL 60548
Elicits specific structures using photographs.
Level I, Ages 3;0–5;0 years and Level II, 5;0–8;0 years

Test for Auditory Comprehension of Language **(TACL),** *Spanish version*
DLM Teaching Resources
One DLM Park
Allen, TX 75002
Tests comprehension of concepts and certain sentence structures.
Ages 3;0–6;0 years

Test de Vocabulario en Imagenes Peabody **(TVIP)**
American Guidance Publishers' Building
Circle Pines, MN 55014
Tests receptive vocabulary.
Ages 2;6–18 years

Toronto Test of Receptive Vocabulary
National Educational Laboratory Publishing
P. O. Box 1003
Austin, TX 78767
Tests receptive vocabulary in Spanish and English using line drawings.
Ages 4;0–10;0 years

Spanish Expressive Vocabulary Test
Los Amigos Research Associates
7035 Galewood
San Diego, CA 92120
(619) 286-3162
Provides an estimate of the child's expressive Spanish vocabulary.
Grades pre-K through 6th

Multicultural Vocabulary Test
Los Amigos Research Associates
7035 Galewood
San Diego, CA 92120
(619) 286-3162

Measures expressive vocabulary development in Spanish-speaking or bilingual children.
Ages 3;0–12;0 years

Prueba del Desarrollo Inicial del Lenguaje (PDIL)
Pro-Ed
8700 Shoal Creek Boulevard
Austin, TX 78757
(512) 451-3246
Tests receptive and expressive language through semantic and syntactic tasks.
Ages 3;0–7;0 years

Preschool Language Assessment Instrument (PLAI)
The Psychological Corporation
Harcourt Brace & Company
555 Academic Court
San Antonio, TX 78204
1-800-228-0752
Identifies children whose language difficulties impede classroom performance.
Ages 2;9–5;8 years

Clinical Evaluation of Language Fundamentals—3 (CELF-3) **Spanish Edition**
The Psychological Corporation
Harcourt Brace & Company
555 Academic Court
San Antonio, TX 78204
1-800-228-0752
Evaluates language development of Spanish-speaking students.
Ages 6;0–21;0 years

Boehm Test of Basic Concepts—Revised
The Psychological Corporation
Harcourt Brace & Company
555 Academic Court
San Antonio, TX 78204
1-800-228-0752
Measures mastery of 50 basic concepts.
Grades kindergarten–2

Bilingual Syntax Measure I and II (**BSM I and BSM II**)
The Psychological Corporation
Harcourt Brace & Company
555 Academic Court
San Antonio, TX 78204

1-800-228-0752
Measures oral proficiency in Spanish
Grades: BSM I- Prekindergarten through grade 2
BSM II-Grades 3–12

Woodcock-Munoz Language Survey
The Riverside Publishing Company
Houghton Mifflin
8420 Bryn Mawr Avenue
Chicago, IL 60631
Screening instrument that aids in decision of ESL placement.
Ages 4;0–adult

***Woodcock Language Proficiency Battery* (WLPB)**
The Riverside Publishing Company
Houghton Mifflin
8420 Bryn Mawr Avenue
Chicago, IL 60631
Measures oral language, written language, and reading.
Ages 4;0–19;11

***Assessment of Children's Language Comprehension* (ACLC)**
The Riverside Publishing Company
Houghton Mifflin
8420 Bryn Mawr Avenue
Chicago, IL 60631
Tests receptive language.
Ages 3;0–6;0

***Receptive One-Word Vocabulary Tests* (ROWPVT), (ROWPVT-Upper Extension)**
The Riverside Publishing Company
Houghton Mifflin
8420 Bryn Mawr Avenue
Chicago, IL 60631
ROWPVT assesses the level of receptive vocabulary development.
Ages 2;0–11;0 years
ROWPVT-UE assesses receptive vocabulary.
Ages 12;0–15;0 years

***Expressive One-Word Picture Vocabulary* (EOWPVT-Revised), (EOWPVT-Upper Extension)**
The Riverside Publishing Company

Houghton Mifflin
8420 Bryn Mawr Avenue
Chicago, IL 60631
EOWPVT-R assesses measures verbal expression of language through association
of words with pictures.
Ages 2;0–11;0 years
EOWPVT-UE assesses expressive vocabulary.
Ages 12;0–15;0 years

Bilingual Vocabulary Assessment Measure
Academic Communication Associates
Publication Center, Dept. 206
4149 Avenida de la Plata
P.O. Box 586249
Oceanside, CA 92058
(619) 758-9593
Assesses expressive bilingual knowledge of basic vocabulary.
Ages 3;0–adult

Spanish Language Assessment Procedures (**SLAP**)
Academic Communication Associates
Publication Center, Dept. 206
4149 Avenida de la Plata
P.O. Box 586249
Oceanside, CA 92058
(619) 758-9593
Assesses the pragmatic and structural aspects of the Spanish language. Includes an
articulation screening instrument.
Ages 3;0–9;0 years

Spanish Test for Assessing Morphologic Production (**STAMP**)
Academic Communication Associates
Publication Center, Dept. 206
4149 Avenida de la Plata
P.O. Box 586249
Oceanside, CA 92058
(619) 758-9593
Assesses production of Spanish morphemes.
Ages 5;0–11;0 years

Dos Amigos Verbal Language Scales
Academic Communication Associates
Publication Center, Dept. 206
4149 Avenida de la Plata

P.O. Box 586249
Oceanside, CA 92058
(619) 758-9593
Measures verbal opposites.
Ages 5;0–13;0 years

Other Tests

Brigance, A. (1983). *Brigance diagnostic assessment of basic skills* (Spanish version). North Billerica, MA: Curriculum Associates.

Compton, A. J., & Kline, M. *Compton speech and language screening evaluation* (Spanish adaptation). San Francisco, CA: Carousel House.

Fenson, L., Dale, P., Rexznick, J. S., Thal, D., Bates, E., hartung, J. P., Pethick, S., Rielly, J. S. *Fundacion MacArthur inventario del desarrollo de habilidades comunicativas,* (Spanish adaptation of the MacArthur Communicative Development Inventory [CDI]). San Diego, CA: University of California, San Diego, Dept. of Psychology.

Hendrick, D.L., Prather, M., & Tobin, A. R. *Sequenced inventory of communication development* (Spanish adaptation). Seattle, WA: University of Washington Press.

Age 0–3
Preschool Language Scale-3
Fundación MacArthur Inventario del Desarrollo de Habilidades Comunicativas
Sequenced Inventory of Communication Development

Preschool (3–5)
Assessment of Phonological Processes
Austin Spanish Articulation Test
Compton speech and language screening evaluation
Del Rio Language Screening Test
Medida Española de Articulacion
Preschool Language Scale—3
Screening Test of Spanish Grammar
Sequenced Inventory of Communication Development
Spanish Articulation Measures
Structured Photographic Elicitation Language Test
Test for Auditory Comprehension of Language
Test de Vocabulario en Imagenes Peabody
Toronto Test of Receptive Vocabulary

Spanish Expressive Vocabulary Test
Multicultural Vocabulary Test
Prueba del Desarrollo Inicial del Lenguaje
Preschool Language Assessment Instrument
Boehm Test of Basic Concepts-Revised
Bilingual Syntax Measure I and II
Woodcock-Muñoz Language Survey
Woodcock Language Proficiency Battery
Assessment of Children's Language Comprehension
Receptive One-Word Vocabulary Test
Expressive One-Word Picture Vocabulary
Bilingual Vocabulary Assessment Measure
Spanish Language Assessment Measure

School Age (5–12)
Brigance Diagnostic Assessment of Basic Skills
Spanish Test for Assessing Morphologic Production
Dos Amigos Verbal Language Scales
Assessment of Phonological Processes
Austin Spanish Articulation Test
Del Rio Language Screening Test
Medida Española de Articulacion
Preschool Language Scale—3
Screening Test of Spanish Grammar
Spanish Articulation Measures
Structured Photographic Elicitation Language Test
Test for Auditory Comprehension of Language
Test de Vocabulario en Imagenes Peabody
Toronto Test of Receptive Vocabulary
Spanish Expressive Vocabulary Test
Multicultural Vocabulary Test
Prueba del Desarrollo Inicial del Lenguaje
Preschool Language Assessment Instrument
Boehm Test of Basic Concepts-Revised
Bilingual Syntax Measure I and II
Woodcock-Muñoz Language Survey
Woodcock Language Proficiency Battery
Assessment of Children's Language Comprehension
Receptive One-Word Vocabulary Test
Expressive One-Word Picture Vocabulary
Bilingual Vocabulary Assessment Measure
Spanish Language Assessment Measure
Clinical Evaluation of Language Fundamentals—3

Adolescent (12–18)
Assessment of Phonological Processes
Spanish Articulation Measures
Test de Vocabulario en Imagenes Peabody
Clinical Evaluation of Language Fundamentals—3
Woodcock-Muñoz Language Survey
Woodcock Language Proficiency Battery
Receptive One-Word Vocabulary Test-Upper Extension
Expressive One-Word Picture Vocabulary-Upper Extension
Bilingual Vocabulary Assessment Measure
Dos Amigos Verbal Language Scales

TREATMENT MATERIALS

Bilingual Speech Source (publisher)
1119 West Webster Ave, Ste 100
Chicago, Illinois 60614
1-800-825-7133

*Una programa de articulacion: El
    sonido /s/*
Los Amigos Research Associates
San Diego, California

*Experiencias en espanol workbook
    and teachers guide*
National Textbook Company
Lincolnwood, Illinois

Signos para el Ingles exacto
Modern Signs Press, Inc.
Los Alamitos, California

Initial sounds in Spanish
Ideal School Supply Company
Oak Lawn, Illinois

*Teaching Spanish speech sounds:
    Drills for articulation therapy*
Academic Communication Associates
Publication Center, Dept. 206
4149 Avenida de la Plata
P.O. Box 586249
Oceanside, CA 92058
(619) 758-9593

APPENDIX

G

English and Spanish Professional Terminology

Terminology	Terminología
Academic Achievement	**Aprovechamiento Escolar** El progreso del niño en sus estudios academicos. La cualidad de trabajo que el estudiante hace. El nivel en cual el estudiante se desarrolla.
Adaptations	**Adaptaciones** Cosas que los maestros hacen para ayudar al estudiante aprender o desarrollarse más en la clase.
Adaptive Techniques	**Tecnicas Adaptativas** Metodos que cada uno usa para adaptarse a las circunstancias.
Adaptive Behavior	**Conductas Adaptativas** Comportamiento que usa uno para adaptarse a la situacíon. La habilidad de un estudiante de hacerse más independiente.

Terminology	*Terminología*
Adaptive Tools	**Estrategía De Adaptacíon** Estrategías que nosotros usamos para ayudar a la persona a adaptarse a la situacíon.
Articulation	**Articulación** La manera de pronunciar las palabras. La manera de como se pronuncian los sonidos del habla. El movimiento de la boca, lengua, dientes, para producir sonidos para hablar.
Assessment	**Evaluacíon** Un serie de exámenes para llegar a un díagnostico. El processo de probar las habilidades del habla y el lenguaje para estableser el nivel de habilidad. Puede incluir exámenes como observaccíones del estudiente, y entrevistas con personas que lo conocen.
Assistive Technology	**La Tecnología De Apoyo** Instrumentos tecnologicos que uno utiliza para communicarse. El uso de la maquina, computadoras, audífonos, tablerors de comunicacíon o cualquier tecnología para facilitar comunicacíon con una persona con deshabilidades.
At-Risk Children	**Niños Con Alto De Deshabilidades Riesgo** El niño está en peligro de no desarrollarse en su nivel adecuando. Niños con determinadas condiciones abientales, médicas, o psicologicas. Los que tendrian un impacto negativo al desarrollo
Audiogram	**Audiograma** Instrumento que enseña el nivel audiologico de la persona. Es una gráfica que enseñar los resultados de la evaluacíon audiologica.
Audiological Evaluation	**Evaluacíon Audiologica** Es un examen que determina el nivel del sentido del oído.
Audiology	**Audiología** El estudio del sentido del oído. Es una evaluación para determinar la habilidad de oído.

Terminology	*Terminología*
Auditory Discrimination	**Distinción Auditiva** La manera en que se distinuen los sonidos en partes de una palabra or una frase. Por ejemplo, se da cuenta de la deferencia en "mesa" y "masa."
Behavior Management Plan	**Plan De Desarrollo Para Manejar la Conducta** Metodos para modificar la conducta del niño.
Borderline	**Fronterizo** La linea divisoria El borde entre dos cosas. Por ejemplo, el niño esta entre el nivel normal y el nivel retrasado.
Brain Lesion	**Lesion Cerebrál** Herida en el cerebro.
Council For Exceptional Children (U.S.)	**Consejo Para Niños Excepcionales** Un concilio para maestros, professionales, y padres de niños excepcionales.
Certification	**Certificación** Documentos que demuestran una especialidad.
Child-Find and Screening	**Ubicación E Identificación De Niños** Una organizacion que identifica y ubica a los niños que necesitan ayuda especial.
Cleft Palate	**Paladar Hendido** Es una condición en que el paladar esta separado de si mismo.
Cognitive Development	**Desarrollo Cognitivo** El desarrollo del la capacidad de la persona (como aprenden, entienden, etc.).
Cognitive Skills	**Habilidades Y Capacidades** Capacidad y disposicíon para pensar. Facilidad de hacer algo de pensamineto o comprención.
Communication Development	**Desarrollo De La Comunicación** Algo que se va haciendo o desarrollando para comunicarse, o hablar con una persona.
Concrete Experiences	**Experiencias Concretas** Algo que hemos realizado en especial. Enseñanza que se adquiere con la practica en resumen o en conclusión.
Consonants	**Consonantes** Letras del alfabeto que no son vocales.

Terminology	*Terminología*
Continuum	**Continuo** Aplicarse a las cosas que tienen union entre si mismo. Algo que se hace sin parar.
Deaf	**Sordo** Que no oye, o no oye bien.
Delays	**Retrasos** Esta referido a un rendimiento intelectual por debajo del promedio general que se manfiesta durante el perirodo de crecomiento de un niño.
Developmentally Appropriate	**Practicas Apropiadas Para El Desarrollo** Practicas de cosas que se hacen para llevar a cabo algun proyecto o plan de desarrollo.
Diagnosis	**Diagnostico** El arte o hecho para determinar la naturaleza de la enfermedad de un paciente. Conclusión alcanzada en la identificacíon de la enfermedad de un paciente.
Dysphagia	**Disfagia** Difficultad o incapacidad para pasar o tragar la comida. **Disfagia Constricta:** Dificultad para la comida a causa de fatiga muscular en el esofago. **Disfagia Espastica:** Dificultad paar pasar los liquidos y no de solidos.
Ear Infection	**Infeccíon Del Oído** Es una enfermad contagiada o producida por un virus o germen. Causa de infeccíon o tiene caracter de tal: enfermedad contagiada de un virus o germen del organo de la audicíon que puede consistir de el oído externo, oido medio o el oído interno o laberinto.
Ear **(Middle, Inner, Outer)**	**Oído** **(Medio, Interno, Externo)** **Oído (Organo De Oido):** Lo que comunmente llamamos la oreja. organo de la audicíon que consiste de oído medio, y oído interno o laberinto. **Oído Externo:** La parte que vemos por fuera.

Terminology	Terminología
	Oído Medio: Estas membranas estan dentro del oído y por lo general nunca las vemos. Cavidad timpanica con extructuras relacionadas, que incluye la membrana timpanica, los osiculos, la trompa auditiva.
	Oído Interno: Laberinto que contiene los organos esenciales del oido.
Early Childhood	**Infancia** La primera etapa de la vida de un niño desde que nace hasta que se combierte en joven.
Early Intervention	**Intervención Temprana** Intervenir antes de que se forme algún problema.
Empower	**Aumentar Potencial** Agregor energia para realizar un proyecto o trabajo.
Enhance	**Acentuar/Aumentar** Recalcar con enfasers o realizar las palabras para dar mas expresíon.
Excessive Nasality	**xceso De Nasalidad** Relativo al exceso de aire que pasa por la naríz al pronunciar palabras.
Fetal Alcohol Syndrome	**Sindrome De Alcoholismo Fetal** Abnormalidades congjnétas causadas al feto por el exceso de consumo de alcohol durante el embarazo.
Fine Motor	**Motor Fino** Se refiere a movimientos, discretos o especiales que requieren el uso de musculos pequeños. Un movimiento pequeño.
Gross Motor	**Motor Grueso o Globales** Se refiere a movimientos grandes que requieren musculos refinados para actividades de locomotor (el poder moverse de un lugar a otro) y equilibro. Un movimiento grande de los extremos (brazos, piernas).
Frenum	**Frenillo** Es la membrana que sujeta la lengua por la linea media de la parte inferior.

Terminology	Terminología
Gestures And Signs	**Gestos Y Señas** Expresíon con que se muestran los diversos estados de animo. Movimiento de cualquije parte del cuerpo para expresar o enfatizár una idea. Movimiento exagerado del rostro por habito o enfermedad.
Goals And Objectives	**Metas Y Objetivos** **Metas:** Fin a que se dirigen las accíones o deseos de una persona. **Objectivos:** Deseos que una persona se propone a realizar.
Hearing Impairment	**Impedimento Auditivo** Obstaculo, estorbo para oír. Algo que impide oír. Abstaculo, estrobo limitando las funcciones del organo de la audicíon.
Hearing Loss	**Perdida De Audicion O Sentido Del Oido**
Higher Order Thinking Skill	**Procesos Ejecutivos** Pensamientos que requieren alto nivel de desarrollo y entendimiento.
Hoarseness	**Ronquera** El sonido que produce una persona cuando la voz se oye ronca.
IQ	**Cociente Intelectual** Las habilidades de tu mente
Individual Education Plan	**Plan Educativo Individual** Determinado programa que se apropia para un niño.
Infant/Toddler	**Infante** Un niño recien nacido de cero a tres años.
Knowledge	**Conocimiento** Desarrollo o sabiduria de una persona.
Language Impairment	**Impedimiento Del Habla** Obstaculo, estorbo limitando las funciones del habla.
Larynx	**Laringe** Organo del sonido de la voz.

Terminology	*Terminología*
Learning Problems	**Problemas De Aprendizaje** Cuando una persona tiene problemas de aprender y entender las cosas académicas.
Learning Disabilities	**Incapacidad De Aprendizaje** Es cuando una persona no puede aprender como otros personas y por eso necesita más ayuda para aprender.
Lesson Plans	**Planes De Clase** Planes de actividades para cada día que tiene metas para ayudar los niños de habla y lenguaje.
Literacy Development	**Desarrollo De La Lectoescritura** Desarrolla de leer y escribir que empieza con nacimiento y continua durante los años
Literacy	**Alfabetización** Es la capacidad de leer y escribir.
Mentally Retarded	**Retrasado Mental** Las habilidades de mente que estan por debajo de lo normal.
Modality	**Modalidad** Modo de ser. Acciones externas con que uno da conocer su buena o mala educacíon.
Moderate Delay	**Retraso Moderado**
Multi-Handicapped	**Con Discapacidades Multiples** Cuando tiene más de un problema ya sea mental o fisico.
Multicultural	**Multicultural** Contiene aspectos de varias culturas.
Muscular Dystrophy	**Distrofia Muscular** La debilidad en los musculos.
National Association Of Bilingual Education	**Asociacíon Nacional Para Las Bilinguajes** Asociación nacional para los profesionales en la educación bilingüe (NABE).
Bilingual Education	**Educacíon Bilingüe**
Neurological Evaluation	**Evaluacion Neurologica**
Occlusions	**Obstrucción** Algo que impide pasar

Terminology	Terminología
Omission (To Omit A Sound)	Omisíon (Dejar De Pronunciar Un Sonido)
Otologist	Otólogo /Aurista Es un especialista del oído que hace estudios diagnosticos y tratamientos de las enfermadades del oído.
Paralysis	Parálisis Es cuando una parte de sus musculos no funcióna y pierde fuerza ó sensación.
Paraplegic	Paraplejico Es una persona que tiene parálisis en las piernas.
Paraprofessionals	Paraprofesionales Es una persona que es un ayudante de un profesional. Por ejemplo, una ayudante de una maestra.
Phonological Disorder	Desorden Fonologico Es cuando niños tienen una sistema de reglas de combinando los sonidos y que es diferente de los niños normales.
Phonological Processes	Procesos Fonologicos Procesos o reglas que encuentran errores de substitución, omisión, o adicíon de combinaciones de sonidos. Por ejemplo, "patano" por "platano."
Physical Development	Desarrollo Físico El desarrollo del cuerpo.
Preschool	Preescolar Antes de kindergarten y los niños tienen 3 a 5 annos de edad.
Problem-Solving	Procesos De Resolucíon De Problemas La habilidade que tiene los procesos que mira un situacíon o problema, y pueden solucionar esa problema.
Psychological Evaluation	Evaluación Psicologíca Es una evaluacíon de la mentales de una persona.
Psychosocial	Psicosocial Relativo a la vida social.
Resource-Room	Cuarto De Apoyo Pedagogico Lugar ofo programa de ayuda al niño.

Terminology	*Terminología*
Screening	**Prueba De Selección**
Screening Process	**Proceso De Detección**
Self-Contained	**Recluido/Auto Contenido** Lugar or programa diseñado para ayudar a niños con ciertas deshabilidades en un ambiente recluido
Social Skills	**Habilidades Sociales**
Socio/Emotional Development	**Desarrollo Social Y Emocional**
Special Education Placement	**Ubicacíon En El Programa De Educacíon Especial**
Speech/Language Delay	**Retraso De Habla Y Lenguaje**
Speech/Language Pathology	**Patología Del Habla Y Lenguaje**
Speech/Language Evaluation	**Evaluación Del Habla Y Lenguaje**
Speech Mechanism	**Mecanismo Del Habla**
Standardized Tests	**Pruebas Estandarizadas** Pruebas diseñadas de materia especifica cuales son administradas a todo tip de niño.
Stutterer	**Tartamudo (A)**
Stuttering	**Tartamudear**
Substitution	**Sustitucion** Reemplazar un sonido por otro
Team	**Equipo (Groupo De Personas)**
Techniques	**Tecnicas** Reglas que se usan para desarrollar y ayudar el niño aprender.
Tonsils	**Amigdalas o Anginas**
Training	**Entrenamiento**
Treatment	**Tratamiento**
Transition	**Transición**
Traumatic Brain Injury	**Lesión o Trauma Al Cerebro**
Visual Discrimination	**Discriminación Visual**

Terminology	Terminología
Visual Impairment	Impedimento Visual Obstaculo o estorbo limitando la vista.
Visual-Motor	Viso-Motriz Movimiento delgado o grueso relativo a la visión.
Velum	Velo Del Paladar Pliege muscular y membranoso suspendido de la parte de atras del paladar.
Vocal Cords	Cuerdas Vocales
Vocal Exercises	Ejercicios Vocales
Vocal Intensity	Intensidad De La Vóz
Vocal Quality	Calidad De La Vóz
Voice	Vóz
Voice (Harsh, Strident, Rough)	Vóz (Aspera, Estridente, Ronco) Aspectos que diserencian el sonido del vóz.
Vowels	Vocales
Whole Language	Lenguaje Integral

APPENDIX

H

Hispanic Holidays

January 6	Three Kings' Day (Traditional)
January 11	Eugenio Maria De Hostos' Birthday (Puerto Rico)
January 18	Jose Mari's Birthday (Cuba)
February 24	Flag Day (Mexico)
February 27	Independence Day (Dominican Republic)
March 21	Benito Juarez' Birthday (Mexico)
March 22	Abolition Day (Puerto Rico)
April 16	Jose De Diego's Birthday (Puerto Rico)
May 1	Dia de Trabajo (Cuba)
May 5	Cinco de Mayo (Mexico)
May 15	Independence Day (Paraguay)
May 19	Jose Marti's Death (Cuba)
May 20	Independence Day (Cuba)

July 5	Independence Day (Venezuela)
July 9	Independence Day (Argentina)
July 17	Munoz Rivera's Birthday (Puerto Rico)
July 20	Independence Day (Columbia)
July 25	Constitution Day (Puerto Rico)
July 27	Jose Celso Barbosa's Birthday (Puerto Rico)
July 28	Independence Day (Peru)
August 6	Independence Day (Bolivia)
August 10	Independence Day (Ecuador)
August 11	Fidel Castro's Birthday (Cuba)
September 15	Independence Day (Nicaragua, Guatemala, Honduras, El Salvador, and Costa Rica)
September 16	Independence Day (Mexico)
September 18	Independence Day (Chile)
October 10	Grito de Baire (Cuba)
November 3	Independence Day (Panama)
November 19	Discovery of Puerto Rico
November 20	Anniversary of Mexican Revolution
November 27	Fusilamiento de Los Siete Estudiantes (Cuba)
December 7	Antonio Marco's Birthday (Cuba)
December 12	Virgen de Guadalupe Day (Traditional)
December 25	Christmas (Traditional)

GLOSSARY

accommodation: Adjusting speech to make oneself understood.

acculturation: The process by which an individual adapts cognitively and emotionally to a new culture, as well as adapting to its communication system.

additive bilingualism: The second language adds to and does not replace the first language.

AIR: American Institutes for Research.

assimilation: A process whereby an individual or group loses the heritage language and culture, which are replaced by the language and culture of the dominant group.

balanced bilingualism: Approximately equal competence in two languages.

barrios: Spanish for neighborhood. Used in the United States for areas where many Latinos live.

basal readers: Reading texts that use simplified vocabulary and syntax and are used in class sets.

BEA: Bilingual Education Act (United States legislation: part of ESEA—see below).

BICS: basic interpersonal communicative skills

big books: Used frequently in whole language classrooms, they are teachers' books that are physically large enough for students to all see and be able to read along with the teacher.

BSM: Bilingual Syntax Measure (attempts to determine the dominant language of a Spanish-English-speaking bilingual).

CALP: cognitive academic language proficiency. The level of language required to understand academically demanding subject matter in a classroom. Such usage is often abstract, lacking contextual supports such as gestures and viewing objects.

caretaker speech: A simplified language used by parents to children to ensure understanding.

Chicanos: An ethnic identity marker for Mexican Americans who view themselves as different from first generation Mexicans.

cloze: Used to determine reading comprehension by having a student supply words that have been systematically deleted from a text.

code-switching: Moving from one language to another, inside a sentence or across sentences.

communicative competence: Proficiency to use a language in everyday conversations. This term accentuates being understood rather than being "correct" in using a language.

compensatory education: *see* **deficit model**

comprehensible input: Language delivered at a level understood by a learner.

core subject: A subject that is of prime importance in the curriculum. In the U.S. the three core subjects are mathematics, English, and science.

CUP: common underlying proficiency (in two languages).

DBE: Dual bilingual education: Also known as two-way bilingual/immersion programs. Two languages are used for approximately equal time in the curriculum.

decoding: In learning to read, the deciphering of the sounds and meanings of letters, combinations of letters, whole words, and sentences of text.

deficit model: The child is perceived as having a language "deficit" that has to be compensated by remedial schooling. The problem is viewed as being in the child rather than in the school system or society or in the ideology of the perceiver. The opposite is an enrichment model (*see* **enrichment bilingual education**).

dialect: A regionally or socially distinctive variety of a language, often with a distinctive pronunciation or accent.

diglossia: Two languages existing together in a society in a stable arrangement through functional distribution.

DL: Dual language (school).

double immersion: Schooling in which subject content is taught through a second and third language (e.g., Hebrew and French for first-language English speakers).

early exit/late exit bilingual education programs: early exit programs move children from bilingual classes in the first or second year of schooling. Late exit programs provide bilingual classes for 3 or more years of elementary schooling. Both programs exist in transitional bilingual education.

EFL: English as a foreign language

equilingual: Someone who is approximately equally competent in two languages.

ESEA: Elementary and Secondary Education Act (United States).

ESOL: English for speakers of other languages.

enrichment bilingual education: develops additive bilingualism, thus enriching a person's life.

ethnocentrism: discriminatory beliefs and behaviors based on the belief that one's own group is superior.

ethnographic pedagogy: Teaching practices and learning strategies derived from ethnography (see below) and conducted in the classroom. An ethnographic researcher becomes involved in a classroom—observes, participates, and helps transform teaching practices.

ethnolinguistic: A set of cultural, ethnic and linguistic features shared by a social group.

ethnography: Study and systematic recording of human cultures, with research that is qualitative rather than quantitative (e.g., engages in fieldwork, interviews, and observation). Such research is often intensive and detailed, hence small-scale.

graphology: The way a language is written.

guest workers: People who are recruited to work in another society or nation. Also known as Gastarbeiter.

hegemony: Domination; the ascendancy of one group over another, expecting compliance and subservience by the subordinate group.

heterogeneous grouping: The use of mixed ability and/or mixed language groups or classes. The opposite is "homogeneous grouping," or tracking (see later).

Hispanics: Spanish speakers in the United States. Official term of the U.S.

immersion bilingual education: Schooling in which some or most subject content is taught through a second, majority language.

in-migrants: Encompasses immigrants, migrants, refugees.

instrumental motivation: Wanting to learn a language for utilitarian reasons (e.g., to get a better job).

integrative motivation: Wanting to learn a language to belong to a social group (e.g., to make friends).

interlanguage: A language integrating aspects of the first and second language used by a second-language learner while learning a second language.

involuntary minorities: Also known as caste-like minorities. They differ from immigrants and "voluntary minorities" in that they have not willingly migrated to a country.

L1/L2: First language, second language.

language minority: A person or a group speaking a language of low prestige or having low numbers in society.

Latinos: Spanish speakers of Latin American extraction. It is the Spanish term which is now used in English, especially by U.S. Spanish speakers, themselves.

LEP: Limited English proficiency.

lexical competency: Competence in vocabulary.

lexis: The vocabulary or word stock of a language.

LMS: Language minority students.

Lingua: A European Community (EC) program to increase majority language learning across Europe. The program funds scholarships, student exchanges, and teaching materials to improve language learning and teaching in the 15 member states of the European Union, plus Iceland, Liechtenstein, and Norway.

lingua franca: A language used between groups of people with different native languages.

linguicism: The use of languages to legitimate and reproduce unequal divisions of power and resources in society.

mainstreaming: Putting a student who has previously been in a special educational program into a regular classroom.

marked language: A minority language distinct from a majority one and usually not highly valued in society.

melting pot: The amalgamation of a variety of immigrant ethnic groups to make a "U.S. American citizen."

OCR: Office of Civil Rights (United States).

parallel teaching: A situation in which bilingual children receive instruction from two teachers working together as a team—each using a different language. The term specifically means a second-language teacher and the classroom teacher planning together, but teaching independently.

phonics: A method of teaching reading based on recognizing the sounds of letters and combinations of letters.

polyglot: Someone competent in several languages.

process instruction: An emphasis on "doing" in the classroom rather than on creating a product. A focus on procedures and techniques rather than on learning outcomes; learning "how to" through inquiry rather than learning through the transmission and memorization of knowledge.

Pygmalion effect: A self-fulfilling prophecy. In a negative mode, a student is labeled (e.g. by a teacher) as having "limited English." The label is internalized by the student who behaves in a way that confirms the label.

racism: A system of privilege and penalty based on race. It is based on a belief in the inherent superiority of one race over others and acceptance of economic, social, political, and educational differences based on such supposed superiority.

reception classes/centers: For newly arriving students.

register: A variety of a language closely associated with different contexts or scenes in which the language is used (e.g., courtroom, classroom, cinema, church) and hence with different people (e.g., police, professor, parent, priest).

remedial bilingual education: Also known as compensatory bilingual education. Uses the native tongue only to "correct" the students' presumed "deficiency" in the majority language.

SAIP: Special alternative instructional programs (United States).

scaffolding approach: Building on a child's existing repertoire of knowledge and understanding.

sheltered English: Content classes with English language development. The teacher uses English that is comprehensible to students but the course content is like that used in other classrooms.

skills-based literacy: Emphasis placed on the acquisition of phonics and other forms, rather than in ways of using those forms.

SL (second language) extension: An option in a secondary school, with the second language allotted extra time on the curriculum. Other students choose different subject options or more time on their first language.

SLT: Second-language teaching.

standard language: A prestige variety of a language (e.g., standard English)

submersion: Schooling that does not allow the child to use his of her home language for learning. The child works solely through a second, majority language.

subtractive bilingualism: The second language replaces the first language.

syntax: Word order. Rules about the ways words are combined.

target language: The language being learned or taught.

TBE: Transitional bilingual education.

TEFL: Teaching English as a foreign language.

TESOL: (a) teachers of English to speakers of other languages; (b) teaching English as a second or other language.

threshold level: A level of language competence a person has to reach to gain benefits from owning two languages.

TPR: Total physical response—method of second language learning.

tracking: The use of homogenous groups (also called setting, streaming, banding, ability grouping).

two-way programs: (*see* **DBE**).

UNESCO: United Nations Educational, Scientific, and Cultural Organization.

vernacular: An indigenous or heritage language of an individual or community.

whole language approach: An amorphous cluster of ideas about language development in the classroom. The approach does not use (is opposed) basal readers (see above) and phonics (see above) in learning to read. Generally, the approach supports a holistic and integrated teaching of reading, writing, spelling, and oracy. The language used must have relevance and meaning to the child. Language development engages cooperative sharing and cultivates empowerment. The use of language for communication is stressed: Function matters rather than the form of language.

REFERENCES

Altenberg, E. P. (1991). Assessing first language vulnerability to attrition. In H. W. Seliger and R. M. Vago (Eds.), *First language attrition* (pp. 189–206). New York: Cambridge University Press.

Ambert, A. N. (1986a). Identifying language disorders in Spanish-speakers. *Journal in Reading, Writing and Learning Disabilities International, 2*(1), 32–41.

Ambert, A. N. (1986b). Identifying language disorders in Spanish-speakers. In A. C. Willig & H. F. Greenberg (Eds.), *Bilingualism and learning disabilities* (pp. 15–36). New York: American Library Publishing Co., Inc.

American Speech-Language-Hearing Association. (1985). Clinical management of communicatively handicapped minority language populations. *Asha 27*(6), 29–32.

American Speech-Language-Hearing Association. (1989). Bilingual speech-language pathologists and audiologists. *Asha, 31*(3), 93.

Anderson, R. T. (1995). Spanish morphological and syntactic development. In H. Kayser (Ed.), *Bilingual speech-language pathology: An Hispanic focus* (pp. 41–74). San Diego: Singular Publishing Group.

Anderson, N. B., & Battle, D. (1993). Cultural diversity in the development of language. In D. Battle (Ed.), *Communication disorders in multicultural populations* (pp. 158–186). Boston: Andover Medical Publishers.

Anderson, P. P., & Fenichel, E. S. P. (1989). *Serving culturally diverse families of infants and toddlers with disabilities.* Washington, DC: National Center for Clinical Infant Programs.

Anderson, R. T. (1996). Assessing the grammar of Spanish-speaking children: A comparison of two procedures. *Language, Speech, and Hearing Services in Schools, 27,* 333–344.

Anderson, R. T. (1997). Examining language loss in bilingual children. *Newsletter of the Special Interest Division: Communication Disorders and Sciences in Culturally and Linguistically Diverse Populations, 3* (pp. 2–5). Rockville, MD: American Speech-Language-Hearing Association.

Baetens-Beardsmore, H. (1982). *Bilingualism: Basic principles.* Boston: College-Hill Press.

Barrera, R. (1997, November). *Insights into U.S. children's English-as-a-second language (ESL) reading.* Presentation at the annual convention of Teachers of Speakers of Other Languages. Orlando, FL.

Beaumont, C. (1992). Language intervention strategies for Hispanic LLD students. In H. Langdon with L. R. L. Cheng (Eds.), *Hispanic children and adults with communi-*

cation disorders: Assessment and intervention (pp. 272–333). Gaithersburg, MD: Aspen Publishers, Inc.

Bernhardt, B., & Stoel-Gammon, C. (1994). Nonlinear phonology: Introduction and clinical application. *Journal of Speech and Hearing Research, 37,* 123–143.

Bernhardt, E. B., & Kamil, M. L. (1998). Literacy instruction of non-native speakers of English. In M. F. Craves, C. Juel, & B. F. Graves (Eds.), *Teaching reading in the 21st century* (pp. 430–475). Boston: Allyn & Bacon.

Bloomfield, L. (1935). *Language.* London: Allen & Unwin.

Brisk, M. R. (1972). *The Spanish syntax of the preschool Spanish-American: The case of New Mexican five-year-old children.* Unpublished dissertation, University of New Mexico.

Brisk, M. R. (1976). The acquisition of Spanish gender by first-grade Spanish-speaking children. In G. D. Keller, R. V. Teschner, & S. Viera (Eds.), *Bilingualism in the bicentennial and beyond* (pp. 143–160). Jamaica, NY: Bilingual Review Press.

Bureau of the Census. (1988, December). Series P-120, 434.

Carrasquillo, A. (1992). A rational for Hispanic representation in instructional materials. *The Journal of Educational Issues of Language Minority Students, 14,* 115–125.

Carrow, E. (1974). *Austin Spanish Articulation Test.* Austin, TX: Learning Concepts.

Chamot, A. (1988). Bilingualism in education and bilingual education: The state of the art in the United States. *Journal of Multilingual and Multicultural Development, 9*(1), 11–35.

Chamot, A. U., & O'Malley, J. M. (1986). *Cognitive/content approach to English language development.* Rosslyn, VA: National Clearinghouse for Bilingual Education.

Cheney, C. (1989). The systematic adaptation of instructional materials and techniques for problem learners. *Academic Therapy, 25*(1), 25–30.

Chesterfield, R., & Chesterfield, K. B. (1985). Natural order in children's use of second language learning strategies. *Applied Linguistics, 6,* 45–59.

Child, I. L. (1943). *Italian or American? The second generation in conflict.* New Haven: Yale University Press.

Corson, D. J. (1990). *Language policy across the curriculum.* Clevedon, England: Multilingual Matters.

Civil Rights Act of 1964, Title VI, Section 601, 42, U.S.C.A., Section 2000d.

Cohen, S. W. (1980). *The sequential order of acquisition of Spanish verb tenses among Spanish-speaking children of age 3–7.* Unpublished doctoral dissertation, University of San Francisco.

Collier, C., & Kalk M. (1989). Bilingual special education curriculum development. In L. Baca & H. T. Cervantes (Eds.), *The bilingual special education interface* (pp. 233–268). Columbus: Merrill.

Conklin, N. F., & Lourie, M. A. (1983). *A host of tongues: Language communities in the United States.* New York: The Free Press.

Corder, S. P. (1967). The significance of learner's errors. *IRAL, 5,* 161–170.

Crawford, J. (1997). *Best evidence: Research foundations of the bilingual education act.* Washington, DC: National Clearinghouse for Bilingual Education.

Cummins, J. (1979). Linguistic interdependence and the educational development of bilingual children. *Review of Educational Research, 49*(2) 221–51.

Cummins, J. (1980). Psychological assessment of immigrant children: Logic or intuition. *Journal of Multilingual and Multicultural Development, 1,* 97–111.

Cummins, J. (1981). The role of primary language development in promoting educational success for language minority students. In *Schooling and language minority students: A theoretical framework* (pp. 1–50). Los Angeles: Evaluation, Dissemination and Assessment Center.

Cummins, J. (1984). *Bilingualism and special education: Issues in assessment and pedagogy.* San Diego: College-Hill Press.

Cummins, J. (1992). Bilingual education and English immersion: The Ramirez report in theoretical perspective. *Bilingual Research Journal, 16,* 1–2, 91–104.

Cummins, J. (1995). Bilingual education and anti-racist education. In O. Garcia & C. Baker (Eds.), *Policy and practice in bilingual education: A reader extending the foundations* (pp. 63–69). Clevedon, England: Multilingual Matters.

Cummins, J. (1996, November). *Negotiating identities: Education for empowerment in a diverse society.* Paper presented at the annual convention of the California Association for Bilingual Education, Ontario, CA.

Dale, P. (1980). *Acquisition of English and Spanish morphological rules by bilinguals.* Unpublished doctoral dissertation, University of Florida, Gainesville.

Damico, J. S., Oller, J. V., Jr., & Storey, M. E. (1983). The diagnosis of language disorders in bilingual children: Surface oriented and pragmatic criteria. *Journal of Speech and Hearing Disorders, 48,* 385–394.

Delgado-Gaitan, C. (1987). Parent perceptions of school: Supportive environments for children. In H. T. Trueba (Ed.), *Success or failure? Learning and language minority student* (pp. 131–155). Cambridge, MA: Newbury House.

Dressler, W. U. (1991). The sociolinguistic and patholinguistic attrition of Breton phonology, morphology, and morphophonology. In H. W. Seliger & R. M Vago (Eds.), *First language attrition* (pp. 99–112). New York: Cambridge University Press.

Education of All Handicapped Children Act of 1975, 20 U.S.C.A., Sections 1411–1420, P.L. 94–142.

Elementary and Secondary Education Act, Title VII (also known as the Bilingual Education Act), Sections *701 et seq.,* 20 U.S.C.A., Sections 880b *et seq.* P. L. 90–247, 81 Stat. 783 (Jan. 2, 1968).

Equal Educational Opportunities Act of 1974, Section 204, 20 U.S.C.A., Section 1703.

Erickson, J. G., & Iglesias, A. (1986). Assessment of communication disorders in non-English proficient children. In O. Taylor (Ed.), *Nature of communication disorders in culturally and linguistically diverse populations* (pp. 181–218). San Diego: College-Hill Press.

Faltis, C. J. (1995). Building bridges between parents and the school. In O. Garcia & C. Baker (Eds.), *Policy and practice in bilingual education: A reader extending the foundations* (pp. 245–258). Clevedon, England: Multilingual Matters.

Fantini, A. E. (1978). *Language acquisition of a bilingual child: A sociolinguistic perspective.* Putney, VT: Experiment Press.

Fillmore, L.W. (1976). *The second time around: Cognitive and social strategies in second language acquisition.* Unpublished doctoral dissertation, Stanford University, Palo Alto, CA.

Fitzgerald, J. (1995, Summer). English-as-a-second-language learners' cognitive reading processes: A review of research in the United States. Review of Education Research.

Fradd, S. H., & Tikunoff, W. J. (1987). *Bilingual education and bilingual special education.* Boston: Little, Brown.

Franklin, S., & Saenz, T. I. (1994, March). *CELF-R modification for bilingual students.* Paper presented at the annual meeting of the California Speech-Language Hearing Association, Sacramento, CA.

Garcia, E. (1988). Effective schooling for language minority students. *Focus, 1,* 1–10.

Garcia, E., & Gonzalez, G. (1984). The interrelationship of Spanish and Spanish/English language acquisition in the Hispanic child. In J. L. Martinez & R. H. Mendoza (Eds.), *Chicano psychology* (2nd ed.) (pp. 427–451). New York: Academic Press.

Garcia E., Maez, L. F., & Gonzalez, G. (1984). *A national study of Spanish-English bilingualism in young Hispanic children of the United States.* Los Angeles: National Dissemination and Assessment Center, California State University.

Garcia, S., & Ortiz, A. (1988). Preventing inappropriate referrals of language minority students to special education. The National Clearinghouse for Bilingual Education. *Occasional Papers in Bilingual Education, 5.*

Garcia Coll, C. T. (1990). Developmental outcome of minority infants: A process-oriented look into our beginnings. *Child Development, 61*(2), 270–289.

Gavillan-Torres, E. (1984). Issues of assessment of limited-English-proficient students and of truly disabled in the United States. In N. Miller (Ed.), *Bilingualism and language disability: Assessment and remediation* (pp. 131–153). San Diego: College-Hill Press.

Genesee, F. (1994). Introduction. In F. Genesee (Ed.), *Educating second language children: The whole child, the whole curriculum the whole community* (pp. 1–12). Cambridge, England: Cambridge University Press.

Genesee, F., & Hamayan, E. V. (1994). Classroom-based assessment. In F. Genesee (Ed.), *Educating second language children: The whole child, the whole curriculum, the whole community* (pp. 212–240). Cambridge, England: Cambridge University Press.

Genishi, C. (1981). Codeswitching in Chicano six-year olds. In R. P. Duran (Ed.), *Latino language and communicative behavior* (pp. 133–152). Norwood, NJ: Ablex Publishers.

Goldstein, B. A. (1995). Spanish phonological development. In H. Kayser (Ed.), *Bilingual speech language pathology: An Hispanic focus* (pp. 17–40). San Diego: Singular Publishing Group.

Goodman, K., Goodman, Y., & Flores, B. (1979). *Reading in the bilingual classroom: Literacy and biliteracy.* Rosslyn, VA: National Clearinghouse for Bilingual Education.

Gonzales, G. (1978). *The acquisition of Spanish grammar by native Spanish-speaking children.* Rosslyn, VA: National Clearinghouse for Bilingual Education.

Gonzalez, G. (1980). *The acquisition of verb tenses and temporal expression in Spanish age 2–4:6.* Bilingual Education Paper Series. Los Angeles: National Dissemination and Assessment Center. California State University.

Gonzalez, G. (1983). Morphology and syntax. In J. Gelett & M. P. Anderson (Eds.), *Bilingual language learning system* (pp. 25–37). Rockville, MD: American Speech-Language-Hearing Association.

Grosjean, F. (1982). *Life with two languages: An introduction to bilingualism.* Cambridge: Harvard University Press.

Gudeman, R. H. (1981). *Learning Spanish: A cross-sectional study of the imitation, comprehension and production of Spanish grammatical forms by rural Panamanians.* Unpublished doctoral dissertation, University of Minnesota, Minneapolis.

Gutierrez-Clellen, V. F. (1995). Narrative development and disorders in Spanish-speaking children: Implications for the bilingual interventionist. In H. Kayser (Ed.), *Bilingual speech-language pathology: An Hispanic focus* (pp. 97–128). San Diego: Singular Publishing Group.

Hakuta, K. (1986). *Mirror of language: The debate on bilingualism.* New York: Basic Books, Inc.

Hakuta, K. (1990). *Bilingualism and bilingual education: A research perspective.* Occasional papers in bilingual education, Number 1. Washington, DC: Office of Bilingual Education and Minority Languages Affairs.

Hanline, M. F., & Daley, S. E. (1992). Family coping strategies and strengths in Hispanic, African-American, and Caucasian families of young children. *Topics in Early Childhood Special Education, 12*(3), 351–366.

Harry, B. (1992). *Cultural diversity, families, and the special education system: Communication and empowerment.* New York: Teachers College Press.

Haugen, E. (1953). *The Norwegian language in America: A study in bilingual behavior.* 2 vols. Philadelphia: University of Pennsylvania Press.

Heath, S. B. (1984, November). *Cross cultural acquisition of language.* Paper presented at the annual convention of the American Speech-Language-Hearing Association, San Francisco.

Heath, S. B. (1986). Social cultural contexts of language development. In *Beyond language: Social and cultural factors in schooling language minority students* (pp. 143–186). Sacramento: California State Department of Education, Bilingual Education Office.

Hodson, B. (1986). *Assessment of phonological processes-Spanish.* San Diego: Los Amigos Association.

Holdaway, D. (1979). *The foundations of literacy.* New York: Ashton Scholastic.

Hoover, J. J., & Collier, C. (1998). Methods and materials for bilingual special education. In L. M. Baca & H. T. Cervantes (Eds.), *The bilingual special education interface* (pp. 264–289). Columbus, OH: Merrill.

Hornak, C., Trujillo, T., & Kayser, H. (1996, November). *Yo sabo Español.* Paper presented at the annual meeting of the American Speech-Language-Hearing Association, Seattle.

Hudelson, S. (1983). Beto at the sugar table: Code switching in the bilingual classroom. In T. H. Escobedo (Ed.), *Early childhood bilingual education* (pp. 31–49). New York: Teachers College.

Hudelson, S. (1985, October). *From MacDonald's to molecules.* Keynote speech. First Annual Southeastern TESOL Conference, Atlanta, GA.

Hudelson, S. (1994). Literacy development of second language children. In F. Genesee (Ed.), *Educating second language children: The whole child, the whole curriculum, the whole community* (pp. 129–158). Cambridge, England: Cambridge University Press.

Iglesias, A. (1978). *Assessment of phonological disabilities.* Unpublished assessment tool, Ohio State University, Columbus.

Johnson, D. M. (1994). Grouping strategies for second language learners. In F. Genesee (Ed.), *Educating second language children: The whole child, the whole curriculum, the whole community* (pp. 183–211). Cambridge, England: Cambridge University Press.

Kaufman, D., & Aranoff, M. (1991). Morphological disintegration and reconstruction in first language attrition. In H. W. Seliger & R. M. Vago (Eds.), *First language attrition* (pp. 175–206). New York: Cambridge University Press.

Kayser, H. (1985). *A study of speech-language pathologists and their Mexican-American language disordered caseloads.* Unpublished doctoral dissertation, New Mexico State University, Las Cruces.

Kayser, H. (1989). Speech and language assessment of Spanish-English speaking children. *Language, Speech, and Hearing Services in Schools, 20,* 226–244.

Kayser, H. (1990). Social communicative behaviors of language-disordered Mexican-American students. *Child Language Teaching Therapy, 6*(3), 255–269.

Kayser, H. (1993). Hispanic cultures. In D. Battle (Ed.), *Communication disorders in multicultural populations* (pp. 114–157). Boston: Andover Medical Publishers.

Kayser, H. (1995a). Assessment of speech and language impairments in bilingual children. In H. Kayser (Ed.) *Bilingual speech-language pathology: An Hispanic focus* (pp. 243–264). San Diego: Singular Publishing Group.

Kayser, H. (1995b). Bilingualism, myths, and language impairments. In H. Kayser (Ed.), *Bilingual speech-language pathology: An Hispanic focus* (pp. 185–206). San Diego: Singular Publishing Group.

Kayser, H., & Restrepo, M. A. (1995). Language samples: Elicitation and analysis. In H. Kayser (Ed.), *Bilingual speech-language pathology: An Hispanic focus,* (pp. 265–288). San Diego: Singular Publishing Group.

Kernan, K., & Blount, B. G. (1966). The acquisition of Spanish grammar by Mexican children. *Anthropological Linguistics, 8,* 1–14.

Kessler, C. (1984). Language acquisition in bilingual children. In N. Miller (Ed.), *Bilingualism and language disability* (pp. 26–54). San Diego: College-Hill Press.

Kiernan, B., & Swisher, L. (1990). The initial learning of novel English words: Two single-subject experiments with minority-language children. *Journal of Speech and Hearing Research, 33,* 707–716.

Lambert, W. E., & Tucker, G. R. (1972). *Bilingual education of children: The St. Lambert experiment.* Rowley, MA: Newbury House.

Langdon, H. W. (1983). Assessment and intervention strategies for the bilingual language disordered student. *Exceptional Children, 50*(1), 37–46.

Langdon, H. W. (1992). *Interpreter/translator process in the educational setting: A resource manual.* Sacramento, CA: Resources in Special Education.

Langdon, H., & Cheng, L. (1992). *Hispanic children and adults with communication disorders.* Gaithersburg, MD: Aspen.

Langdon, H.W., & Saenz, T. I. (1996). *Language assessment and intervention with multicultural students.* Oceanside, CA: Academic Communication Associates.

Laosa, L. M. (1978). Maternal teaching strategies in Chicano families of varied educational and socioeconomic levels. *Child Development, 49,* 1129–1135.

Larsen-Freeman, D. (1986). *Techniques and principles in language teaching.* New York: Oxford University.

Lau v. Nichols, 414 U.S. 563, 94 s. Ct. 786, 39 L.Ed. 2d 1 (1974).

Lee, L. L. (1974). *Developmental sentence analysis.* Evanston, IL: Northwestern University Press.

Leopold, W. F. (1949). *Speech development of a bilingual child: A linguist's record.* 4 vols. Evanston: Northwestern University Press.

Linares-Orama, N., & Sanders, L. J. (1977). Evaluation of syntax in three-year old Spanish-speaking Puerto Rican children. *Journal of Speech and Hearing Research, 20*(2), 350–357.

Lopez, N., Cheng, L., & Kayser, H. (1995). *Norm-reference tests with culturally and linguistically diverse populations*. Paper presented at the annual meeting of the New York Speech-Language-Hearing Association. Albany.

MacNamara, J. (1967). The bilingual's linguistic performance: A psychological overview. *Journal of Social Issues, 23,* 2.

Maestas, A. G., & Erickson, J. G. (1992). Mexican immigrant mothers' beliefs about disabilities. *American Journal of Speech-Language Pathology, 1*(4), 5–10.

Maez, L. F. (1983). The acquisition of nouns and verbs morphology in 18–24 month old Spanish-speaking children. *National Association for Bilingual Education Journal, 7,* 53–68.

Maher, J. (1991). A crosslinguistic study of language contact and language attrition. In H. W. Seliger & R. M. Vago (Eds.), *First language attrition* (pp. 67–84). New York: Cambridge University Press.

Major, R. C. (1992). Losing English as first language. *The Modern Language Journal, 76,* 190–209.

Maldonado, E. (1984). *Profiles of Hispanic students placed in speech, hearing, and language programs in a selected school district in Texas*. Unpublished doctoral dissertation, University of Texas at Austin.

Mann, D. M., & Hodson, B. W. (1992). Spanish-speaking children's phonologies: Assessment and remediation of disorders. *Seminars in Speech and Language, 15*(2) 137–148.

Mattes, L. J., & Omark, D. R. (1991). *Speech and language assessment for the bilingual handicapped* (2nd ed.) Oceanside, CA: Academic Communication Associates.

Maybin, J. (1985). *Working towards a school language policy. In every child's language: An in-service pack for primary teachers* (pp. 95–108). Clevedon, England: Open University and Multilingual Matters.

McCloskey, N., & Schaar, J. H. (1965). Psychological dimensions of anomy. *American Sociological Review, 30,* 14–40.

McClure, E. (1977). Aspects of code-switching in the discourse of bilingual Mexican-American children. In M. Saville-Troike (Ed.), *Linguistics and anthropology. Georgetown university round table on languages and linguistics 1977* (pp. 93–115). Washington, DC: Georgetown University Press.

McLaughlin, B. (1984a). Early bilingualism: Methodological and theoretical issues. In M. Paradis (Ed.), *Early bilingualism and child development* (pp. 19–45). Lisse: Swets and Zeitlinger.

McLaughlin, B. (1984b). *Second-language acquisition in childhood: Vol. 1 preschool children* (2nd ed.). Hillsdale, NJ: Lawrence Erlbaum.

McLaughlin, B. (1985c). *Second-language acquisition in childhood: Vol 2. School-age children* (2nd ed.). Hillsdale, NJ: Lawrence Erlbaum.

Meitus, I. J., & Weinburg, B. (1983). *Diagnosis in speech-language pathology*. Baltimore: University Park Press.

Merino, B. J. (1976). *Language acquisition in bilingual children: Aspects of syntactic development in English and Spanish by Chicano children in grades K–4*. Unpublished doctoral dissertation, Stanford University, Palo Alto, CA.

Merino, B. (1983). Language development in normal and language handicapped Spanish speaking children. *Hispanic Journal of Behavioral Sciences, 5*(4), 379–400.

Merino, B. J. (1992). Acquisition of syntactic and phonological features in Spanish. In H. W. Langdon & L. L. Cheng (Eds.), *Hispanic children and adults with communication disorders* (pp. 57–98). Gaithersburg, MD: Aspen Publishers, Inc.

Met, M. (1994). Literacy development of second language children. In F. Genesee (Ed.), *Educating second language children: The whole child, the whole curriculum, the whole community.* Cambridge, England: Cambridge University Press.

Meyerson, M. D. (1983). Genetic counseling for families of Chicano children with birth defects. In D. R. Omark & J. G. Erickson (Eds.), *The bilingual exceptional child* (pp. 285–300). San Diego: Los Amigos Research Associates.

Miller, J. (1981). *Assessing language production in children.* Baltimore: University Park Press.

Miller, N. (1984). *Bilingualism and language disability: Assessment and remediation.* San Diego: College-Hill Press.

Ogbu, J. (1983). Minority status and schooling in plural societies. *Comparative Education Review, 27*(2), 168–190.

Olarte, G. (1985). *Acquisition of Spanish morphemes by monolingual, monocultural Spanish-speaking children.* Unpublished doctoral dissertation, University of Florida, Gainesville.

Olson, P. (1991). *Referring language minority students to special education.* Washington, DC: Center for Applied Linguistics. (ERIC Clearing House on Languages and Linguistics)

Omark, D. R. (1981). Pragmatics and ethological techniques for the observational assessment of children's communicative abilities. In J. G. Erickson & D. R. Omark (Eds.), *Communication assessment of the bilingual, bicultural child: Issues and guidelines* (pp. 249–284). Baltimore: University Park Press.

Ortiz, A. A. (1984, Spring). Choosing the language of instruction for exceptional bilingual children. *Teaching Exceptional Children, 208–212.*

Ortiz, A., & Maldonado-Colon, E. (1986). Reducing inappropriate referrals of language minority students in special education. In A. C. Willig & H. F. Greenberg (Eds.), *Bilingualism and learning disabilities* (pp. 37–52). New York: American Library.

Ovando, C. J., & Collier, V. P. (1998). *Bilingual and ESL classrooms: Teaching in multicultural contexts.* Boston: McGraw-Hill.

Parra, R. (1982). *The sequential order of acquisition of categories of Spanish adjectives by Spanish-speaking children of age 2 to 12 years.* Unpublished doctoral dissertation, University of San Francisco.

Paulson, D. M. (1991). *Phonological systems of Spanish-speaking Texas preschoolers.* Unpublished master's thesis. Texas Christian University, Fort Worth.

Peña, E., Quinn, R., & Iglesias, A. (1992). The application of dynamic methods to language assessment: A nonbiased procedure. *The Journal of Special Education, 26*(3), 269–280.

Peregoy, S. F., & Boyle, O. F. (1993). *Reading, writing, and learning in ESL: A resource book for K–8 teachers.* White Plains, NY: Longman.

Perozzi, J. A. (1985). A pilot study of language facilitation for bilingual, language handicapped children: Theoretical and intervention implications. *Journal of Speech and Hearing Disorders, 50,* 403–406.

Perozzi, J., & Sanchez, M. (1992). The effect of instruction in L1 on receptive acquisition of L2 for bilingual children with language delay. *Language, Speech, and Hearing Services in Schools, 23,* 348–352.

Peters-Mink, A. (1977). Language learning strategies: Does the whole equal the sum of the parts? *Language, 53,* 560–573.

Ramirez, J. D., Yuen, S. D., Ramey, D. R., Pasta, D. J., & Billings, D. K. (1991). *Final report: Longitudinal study of structured immersion strategy, early-exit, and late-exit transitional bilingual education programs for language-minority children. Executive summary.* San Mateo, CA: Aguirre International.

Ramirez, M., & Castañeda, A. (1974). *Cultural democracy, bicognitive development and education.* New York: Academic Press.

Restrepo, M. (1995). *Identifiers of Spanish speaking children with language impairment who are learning English as a second language.* Unpublished doctoral dissertation, University of Arizona, Tucson.

Reynolds, M. (1984). Classification of students with handicaps. In E. W. Gordon (Ed.), *Review of research in education* (pp. 63–92). Washington, DC: American Educational Research Association.

Romero, M. (1985). *Verb acquisition in Spanish as a native language in Puerto Rico.* Unpublished doctoral dissertation, New York University, New York.

Roseberry, C. A., & Connell, P. J. (1991). The use of an invented language rule in the differentiation of normal and language-impaired Spanish-speaking children. *Journal of Speech and Hearing Research, 34,* 596–603.

Roseberry-McKibbin, C. (1995). *Multicultural students with special language needs: Practical strategies for assessment and intervention.* Oceanside, CA: Academic Communication Associates.

Roseberry-McKibbin, C. (1995). Distinguishing language difference from language disorder in linguistically and culturally diverse students. *Multicultural Education, 4,* 12–16.

Sanchez, R. (1983). *Chicano discourse.* Rowley, MA: Newbury House Publishers.

Scarcella, R. (1990). *Teaching language minority students in the multicultural classroom.* Englewood Cliffs, NJ: Prentice-Hall.

Schiff-Myers, N. B. (1992). Considering arrested language development and language loss in assessment of second language learners. *Language, Speech, and Hearing Services in the Schools, 23,* 28–33.

Silva-Corvalan, C. (1991). Spanish language attrition in a contact situation with English. In H. W. Seliger & R. M. Vago (Eds.), *First language attrition* (pp. 152–171). New York: Cambridge University Press.

Skutnabb-Kangas, T. (1995). Multilingualism and the education of minority children. In O. Garcia & C. Baker (Eds.), *Policy and practice in bilingual education: A reader extending the foundations* (pp. 40–62). Philadelphia: Multilingual Matters.

Snyder-McLean, L., & McLean, J. (1978). Verbal information gathering strategies: The child's use of language to acquire language. *Journal of Speech and Hearing Disorders, 43,* 306–325.

Statistical abstract of the United States. (1991). 111th ed. Washington, DC: U.S. Bureau of the Census; No. 1434

Stoel-Gammon, C., & Dunn, C. (1985). *Normal and disordered phonology in children.* Baltimore: University Park Press.

Stockwell, R. P. (1965). *The sounds of English and Spanish.* Chicago, IL: The University of Chicago Press.

Sutton, C. (1989). Helping the nonnative English speaker with reading. *The Reading Teacher,* 684–688.

Swain, M., & Barik, H. (1978). Bilingual education in Canada: French and English. In B. Spolsky & R. L. Cooper (Eds.), *Case studies in bilingual education* (pp. 22–71). Rowley, MA: Newbury House.

Taylor, O. (1986). Historical perspectives and conceptual framework. In O. Taylor (Ed.), *Nature of communication disorders in culturally and linguistically diverse populations* (pp. 1–18) San Diego: College-Hill Press.

Taylor, O. (1992). *Research designs and methodologies that NIDCD should encourage and support for intramural and extramural research on people of color.* Paper presented to the Working Group: Research and Research Training Needs of Minority Persons and Minority Health Issues, National Institute on Deafness and other Communication Disorders, National Institutes of Health. Bethesda, MD.

Thiery, C. (1976). Le bilinguisme vrai. *Etudes de Linguistique Appliquee, 24,* 52–63.

Toronto, A. S. (1976). Developmental assessment of Spanish grammar. *Journal of Speech and Hearing Disorders, 41,* 150–171.

Toronto, A. (1977). *Southwestern Spanish Articulation Test.* Austin, TX: National Education Laboratory Publishers.

Torres-Guzman, M.E. (1995). Recasting frames: Latino parent involvement. In O. Garcia & C. Baker (Eds.), *Policy and practice in bilingual education: A reader extending the foundations* (pp. 259–272). Clevedon, England: Multilingual Matters.

Turian, D., & Altenberg, E. P. (1991). Compensatory strategies of child first language attrition. In H. W. Seliger & R. M. Vago, (Eds.), *First language attrition* (pp. 207–226). New York: Cambridge University Press.

U.S. Bureau of the Census. (1996). *Statistical abstract of the United States* (116th ed.). Washington, DC: U.S. Bureau of the Census.

U.S. Office for Civil Rights, May 25, 1970, Interpretation of Civil Rights Act, *Federal Register 35,* 11595.

Valdes, G. (1986). *Brothers and sisters: A closer look at the development of cooperative social orientation in Mexican-American children.* Presented at the 37th Annual Convention of the California Association of School Psychologists. Oakland, CA.

Valdes-Fallis, G. (1978). Code switching and the classroom teacher. *Language in education: Theory and practice* (Vol. 4). Arlington, VA: Center for Applied Linguistics.

Vincent, L. J. (1992). *Families and early intervention: Diversity and competence.* (A keynote address delivered at the Division for Early Childhood annual conference in St. Louis, Missouri—Nov. 14, 1991.) *Journal of Early Intervention, 16*(2), 166–172.

Volterra, V., & Taeschner, T. (1978). The acquisition and development of language by a bilingual child. *Journal of Child Language, 5,* 311–326.

Wong-Fillmore, L. (1989). Teachability and second language acquisition. In M. L. Rice & R. L. Schiefelbusch (Eds.), *The teachability of language* (pp. 311–323). Baltimore: Paul H. Brookes Publishing Co.

Wong-Fillmore, L. (1979). Individual differences in second language acquisition. In C. Fillmore, D. Kempler, & W. S. Y. Wang (Eds.), *Individual differences in language ability and language behavior* (pp. 203–228). New York: Academic Press, Inc.

Zayas, L. H., & Palleja, J. (1988). Puerto Rican families: Consideration for family therapy. *Family Relations, 37,* 260–264.

Zehler, A. (1994). Working with English language learners: Strategies for elementary and middle school teachers. Program Information guide, No. 19. Rosslyn, VA: National Clearinghouse for Bilingual Education.

Zentella, A. (1981). Ta bien, you could answer me en cualquier idioma: Puerto Rican code-switching in bilingual classrooms. In R. Duran (Ed.), *Latino language and communicative behavior* (pp. 109–131). Norwood, NJ: Ablex Publishing.

Further Resources for Reading and ESL Students

Ada, A. F. (1987). *A children's literature-based whole language approach to creative reading and writing.* Northvale, NJ: Santillana.

Arnberg, L. (1987). *Raising children bilingually: The pre-school years.* Clevedon, England: Multilingual Matters.

Baker, C. (1995). *A parents' and teachers' guide to bilingualism.* Philadelphia: Multilingual Matters.

Barrera, R. (1983). Bilingual reading in the primary grades: Some questions about questionable views and practices. In T. H. Escobedo (Ed.), *Early childhood bilingual education: A Hispanic perspective* (pp. 164–84). New York: Teachers College.

Bialystok, E., & Hakuta, K. (1994). *In other words: The science and psychology of second-language acquisition.* New York: Basic Books.

Crystal, D. (1986). *Listen to your child: A parent's guide to children's language.* New York: Penguin Books.

De Jong, E. (1986). *The bilingual experience: A book for parents.* Cambridge: Cambridge University Press.

Edelsky, C. (1986). *Writing in a bilingual program: Habia una vez.* Norwood, NJ: Ablex.

Fishman, J. A., & Lovas, J. (1972). Bilingual education in a sociolinguistic perspective. In B. Spolsky (Ed), *The language education of minority children* (pp. 83–93). Rowley, MA: Newbury House.

Hakuta, K. (1986). *Mirror of language: The debate on bilingualism.* New York: Basic Books.

Harding, E., & Riley, P. (1986). *The bilingual family: A handbook for parents.* Cambridge, England: Cambridge University Press.

Hornberger, N. (1991). Extending enrichment bilingual education: Revisiting typologies and redirecting policy. In O. Garcia (Ed.), *Bilingual education: Focus shift in honor of Joshua A. Fishman* (pp. 215–234). Amsterdam: John Benjamins.

Perez, B., & Torres-Guzman, M. (1992). *Learning in two worlds: An integrated Spanish/English biliteracy approach.* New York: Longman.

INDEX